Sex Role Attitudes
and Cultural Change

PRIORITY ISSUES IN MENTAL HEALTH

A book series published under the auspices of
The World Federation for Mental Health

VOLUME 3

Sex Role Attitudes and Cultural Change

Edited by

IRA GROSS

Dept. of Psychology, University of Rhode Island

JOHN DOWNING

Dept. of Psychology, University of Victoria

and

ADMA D'HEURLE

Mercy College, Dobbs Ferry, New York

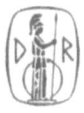

D. REIDEL PUBLISHING COMPANY

DORDRECHT : HOLLAND / BOSTON : U.S.A.

LONDON : ENGLAND

Library of Congress Cataloging in Publication Data

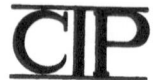

Main entry under title:

Sex role attitudes and cultural change.

(Priority issues in mental health ; v. 3)
Includes index.
1. Sex role—Congresses. 2. Children—Attitudes—
Congresses. 3. Child mental health—Congresses. 4. Social
Change—Congresses. I. Gross, Ira, 1933–   II. Downing,
John A. III. d'Heurle, Adma. IV. Series. [DNLM: 1. Gender
identity. 2. Culture. W1 PR524R v. 3 / WS 105.5.P3 S517]
HQ1075.S48   305.3   81–17805
                                   AACR2

ISBN-13: 978-94-009-7739-6   e-ISBN-13: 978-94-009-7737-2
DOI:10.1007/ 978-94-009-7737-2

Published by D. Reidel Publishing Company,
P.O. Box 17, 3300 AA Dordrecht, Holland.

Sold and distributed in the U.S.A. and Canada
by Kluwer Boston Inc.
190 Old Derby Street, Hingham, MA 02043, U.S.A.

In all other countries, sold and distributed
by Kluwer Academic Publishers Group,
P.O. Box 322, 3300 AH Dordrecht, Holland

D. Reidel Publishing Company is a member of the Kluwer Group

TABLE OF CONTENTS

PREFACE

The initial impetus for this volume was the occasion of the World Congress for Mental Health held in Vancouver, British Columbia in 1977. The theme of that congress was priorities in mental health. The keynote speaker Mrs. Rosalynn Carter, wife of the then President of the United States, focused attention on the necessity for an international perspective in understanding priorities for mental health. Without exception subsequent speakers echoed the sentiments Mrs. Carter expressed, that the first priority for mental health was that of children.

For many participants the concern for children was translated not only into techniques for treatment but more importantly into broadening the approaches to prevention. One theme emerged which has begun to be addressed around the world — that of the cultural and developmental implications of sex role stereotyping for mental health. This topic proved to be the touchstone for many issues related both directly and indirectly to mental health. Among the most prominent concerns expressed were those for the effects on careers, the learning environment and relations between the sexes which stem from stereotyped attitudes concerning appropriate sex role behavior. The consensus of the participants was to urge the directorate of the congress to continue this topic at the next World Congress. This was a particularly appropriate content for the next World Congress, since 1979 was the International Year of the Child.

The subsequent venue in Salzburg brought together the nucleus of participants from the previous World Congress complemented by many others who contributed to a diverse international perspective. This world view disclosed not only the diversity of opinions but the very real dilemma posed by a desire to preserve continuity between prevailing practices on the one hand and the press for change on the other, while preventing the perpetuation of the negative consequences of inappropriate sex role stereotyping.

University of Rhode Island   IRA GROSS, Ph.D.

IRA GROSS, Ph.D.

INTRODUCTION AND OVERVIEW*

The topic of these workshops, "sex role attitudes and cultural change", encompasses diverse issues and approaches from widely differing cultural perspectives. This diversity aroused considerable debate among the participants and served to underscore the vitality of the topic.

Several themes recurred across the topics and these deserve special emphasis:

(1) The existing stereotypes limit the options for behavior of males and females throughout the life cycle. Such constraints violate individual needs for self-actualization and they threaten mental health.

(2) Social agents influence children's attitudes and behavior in many settings. In order for change to occur sex role attitudes must be brought into greater awareness in schools, home, and the community.

(3) Existing knowledge may not yet be wholly adequate for understanding all the implications for changes in attitudes. However, despite the evident shortcomings in our knowledge, there does exist a substantial body of valid information which provides some direction for change. For example, in the family the practice of nonsexist childrearing can encourage positive mental health. Furthermore, the school could introduce curricular materials to encourage nonsexist thinking. More generally, language, which both reflects and affects thinking, could itself be changed to create greater cognizance of healthy attitudes.

The remainder of this chapter will focus on common themes from the content of the workshop papers. We will comment on them and relate them, as appropriate, to the topic of mental health.

I. CROSS CULTURAL PERSPECTIVES ON MENTAL HEALTH AND SEX ROLE SOCIALIZATION

The workshop participants represented a wide diversity of opinions and approaches to research, as well as cultural perspectives. Many of the presentations evoked lively debate. For instance, Dennis Ugwuegbu's interpretation of healthy sex role attitudes ran counter to some of the feminist concerns. He stated that polygyny, a traditional practice in Nigeria, was rejected by the educated elite. His research was directed toward fostering more positive attitudes towards the educated in his country. He was concerned that traditional cultural values and practices in developing countries were being eroded. While the concern for dilution of culture may be genuine, it appeared to other workshop participants that his research perpetuated roles for women which were limiting and regressive. A lively exchange emphasized the fact that not only can we experience a clash

1

I. Gross, J. Downing, and A. d'Heurle (eds.), Sex Role Attitudes and Cultural Change, 1–9.
Copyright © 1982 by D. Reidel Publishing Company.

between modern thinking and traditional values in developing nations, but that, as professionals from different cultures, we must be more finely attuned to each other's needs. For example, some Nigerians relate the changes in marriage patterns to the reduced rate of population growth among the educated elite; this is offered as a reason to encourage polygyny. Despite this argument, the majority of workshop participants concluded that population imbalances between the educated and noneducated should not be redressed by reverting to practices considered psychologically harmful to women.

Differences of opinion regarding culture and change were expressed elsewhere in the workshop. These differences did not seem to come from a lack of appreciation of the respective cultures discussed but, rather, from fundamental differences in interpretation of ideas related to mental health. Thus, while the participants deplored the stereotypes expressed in differential treatment of boys and girls from birth some discussants did not believe there was sufficient scientific knowledge regarding sex role socialization to justify social policy changes. This opinion was roundly debated, with Corinne Hutt stating that there was no evidence to indicate that any policy making body had ever take cognizance of the findings of social science in order to introduce change in its society, anyway.

In addition to some of the theoretical presentations, there were many original empirical studies discussed. Pirkko Niemelä and Rama Pandey focused attention on findings that indicate social change in sex role attitudes and behavior. Dr. Niemelä's study of mothering in Finland yielded evidence that mothers who idealize motherhood provide less healthy role models for their child's behavior than the less traditional mothers. The "idealizing" mothers were much more restricted in their behavioral repertoire and presented fewer alternatives for expression of creative human functioning. They are the very women who choose the traditional exclusionary role of mother and do not seek to actualize themselves in broader personal or vocational ways. As transmitters of culture, it appears that such women do not contribute positively to the mental health of their children because of their rigid adherence to tradition.

Dr. Pandey echoed some of Dr. Niemelä's findings by suggesting that even among the respondents in his study who identified themselves as representing social modernity in India there were those who were contradictory in their value systems. This was evident in their lack of commitment to marriage, education, and occupation while traditional segregation between the sexes still prevails. Nonetheless, the point which he held in common with Dr. Niemelä was that modernization reflects freedom of choice and a degree of flexibility in behavior absent in those who represent more traditional values.

The theme of choice and flexibility in attitudes and behavior was further extended through Susan's Bram's presentation of her research with voluntarily childless couples. Dr. Bram found that the trend toward childlessness is extending beyond the professional middle class in the U.S. and Western Europe, and has begun to include minorities in American society. Thus, it is apparent that childlessness has become a viable alternative although the reasons may not be identical in each social group. The reasons offered by her American sample tend to be proactive, i.e., the desire for personal actualization through a career or an avocation, and not reactive, i.e., based on an aversion to children. Furthermore, the decision reflects a weighing of both the economic and personal costs of parenthood to the wife, the husband, and the couple. It appears that more is at issue in such decision making than simply a question of preferential roles. The data indicates that the choice of childlessness or parenthood reflects a response to the conflict between achievement and affiliative needs which were expressed indirectly in the past, and are now discussed more openly.

Sophia Leung[1] reported that attitudes towards sex roles in the People's Republic of China have become less polarized among young people. She found that decisions regarding career choice and marriage were much more alike than different for men and women. Women were electing to delay marriage for pursuit of a vocation and in many cases their choices for a career were similar to those of men. Women were entering most spheres of work formerly reserved exclusively for men.

Adma d'Heurle reviewed the evolution of sex role perceptions in the cinema of François Truffaut and illustrated the social concern for this issue. The image of the traditional separation of romantic love from lust has given way to a new image of woman's role in the cinema and thus indicates the need for a new dialectic of love. The woman can no longer be described as an object to be molded by her male partner. In this new image of woman she begins to assert a more active role in defining herself. Surely, this need for self-definition is a natural extension of the idea encountered in the presentations of this workshop which emphasize the idea of conscious choice, awareness and hence a positive expression of self-actualization all of which are concomitants of mental health.

II. ENVIRONMENTAL INFLUENCE ON THE ACQUISITION OF SEX ROLES: PARENTS, TEACHERS, AND LANGUAGE

The theme of awareness and the need to delineate and control the forces which shape sex roles was nowhere more apparent than in the papers contained in this section. The concern which they express regarding environmental influences on the processes by which those roles are acquired ranged across diverse aspects of society. The scope of these topics included early experiences within the family and the attitudes parents convey to their children; differential health care for boys and girls; the role of the school in attitude formation; and development of curricular materials to be used in guiding healthy sex role development.

It is quite apparent that sex role development, like other aspects of a child's formation of skills and character, does not emerge from a neutral background. The social forces and their influence evoked professional concern among workshop participants and incited often lively debate regarding the very nature of these forces.

Ira Gross expressed his concern in several ways, starting with the deficiencies of existing theories of development. Not the least among the problems with existing theory is the fact that it is far from neutral in its interpretation of the ways in which behavior develops. What is disturbing is the lack of awareness by theoreticians of the origins of bias in their thinking about developmental theory in general and specifically about sex role development. At times these theories reflect a male elitism which, historically, derives from status differences between the sexes. One antidote for such nonsconscious bias might be to introduce a dialogue at several levels, such as that generated at this workshop. Furthermore, it is equally important that other agents engaged in socialization, such as schools and parents, also engage in a process of self review and consciousness-raising.

The role of the school in the United States for encouraging equal opportunity for the sexes has been limited to reactions to federal legislation, as Carol Dwyer reported. This has not brought with it a comparable concern by teachers and administrators for the impact of their attitudes on sex role learning. Another step is needed to reduce the dissonance between legal compliance and attitudes which perpetuate narrow, outdated stereotypes. Without the essential element of attitude change, genuine social change is unlikely.

The effects of the schools are transmitted in ways other than the attitudes of educators. The very materials and curricular designs contribute to the inculcation of sex role attitudes and behavior. I. Kallab, J. Abu Nasr, and I. Lorfing examined the role of textbooks in conveying and maintaining traditional stereotypes. They reviewed Arab texts and found that they reinforce the cultural message regarding the role appropriate for women in Lebanese society. Their results corroborate those found in surveys on the content of European and American textbooks. Basically, the female is described in restricted roles as the nurturant figure in the home, self-sacrificing and without personal identity. The polarized image of male and female roles does not reflect the social reality in any of these cultures. For example, Lebanese women have entered the previously exclusive domains of men by attending universities and entering the labor market. The authors deplore the absence of texts which model the new image of men as well as women in more realistic representations. Beyond this they were concerned that the inspirational nature of the texts lost the opportunity to encourage more dynamic roles for women. They implore the writers of texts to consider their responsibility for altering the traditional image of women.

In a similar vein Selma Hughes considered the existing literature on non-sexist curricula and analyzed its contribution to educational change. She introduced several cautionary observations regarding the quality of programs and material. Her concerns derive from the fact that there is a lack of consensus about criteria for the design, and evaluation of curricula. Perhaps the most positive outcome to be expected at this time from efforts at introducing change in the schools is that school personnel will be alerted to the issues they must themselves confront simultaneously with their facilitation of the search for healthy sex roles in boys and girls. Among the suggestions her review identified were the need to develop competence in school age children through their recognition and expression of feelings regardless of sex. While schools may still be sorting out their role as initiators of change, in society at large the debate about sex roles and health will continue to progress around, and often in, the school.

A further contribution to our expanding concern for sex role stereotypes was made in the area of language usage. As a carrier of culture and a transformer of ideas, language is a powerful instrument for conveying messages which may be nonconscious. Shirley Ernst clarified the significant role language has played throughout human history in manipulating people, defining them, and often deciding their fates. In some instances, a whole nation may be destroyed when language distorts reality. In the instance of women it may be their humanity which is destroyed through the stereotyping perpetuated by language bias. The values of a society are actively transmitted through language and impinge upon decisions regarding prescribed and proscribed roles, aspirations, and expectations in life. Regardless of the manner in which stereotypes may originate, it is language which holds up a mirror for society to view its values and attitudes. Ernst suggests that if we desist in using language as a tool for sex role stereotyping, this will greatly contribute to a revision in the selection of role behavior along more appropriate dimensions than gender. Currently, the overriding influence of language seems to be in its exclusionary use. Whatever its contribution may prove to be, it is certain that language can mediate change as well as reflect it.

III. THE INFLUENCE OF SEX ROLE ATTITUDES ON CHILDREN'S ASPIRATIONS

That sex roles affect the greater part of an individual's essential decisions in life has been made abundantly clear. While the manner in which such decisions come to be affected has not yet been clarified in the same ways as its effects there have been some tentative suggestions about their workings. Certainly they make their presence known early in life. Sophia Leung and Betty Kleinman found that as early as four years of age first generation Canadians from three different ethnic origins all had an awareness of sex roles, with males demonstrating a more clearly defined stereotypic notion of the masculine role. Their findings corroborate the results of earlier research efforts. They do not, however, speak to the issue of reasons for the presence of this finding in males. Certainly, as was suggested in the workshop discussion, it is quite possible that the more detailed articulation of masculinity may derive from several sources. For instance, the fact that masculine roles are often reinforced as "good" may contribute to the earlier espousal of these roles by boys.

The earlier, more rigidly defined development of sex roles for boys may have some correlates in school performance. John Downing and Alice Gross, respectively, point to the overrepresentation of boys in clinics and special reading programs. Alice Gross suggested that the sex role definition may contribute to the prevalence of male dyslexia. Despite the evidence supporting social theories of dyslexia the past has borne witness to the almost exclusive attribution to male biological vulnerability. Theories of biological vulnerability have been employed to account for many other dysfunctional behavior in males. Among those behaviors relevant for schooling which have been most intensively researched, reading has a preeminent position as a topic of concern throughout this century. In her research in Israel, Dr. Gross's comparisons of the kibbutz and other communities do not lend support to a biological interpretation. On the contrary, her findings on the kibbutz intimate that equalization of sex role socialization eliminates the vast difference in incidence of dyslexia between boys and girls. Dr. Downing emphasizes the fact that nonconscious attitudes toward sex role often makes accessibility to literacy differentially available to either sex. Most importantly he rivets our attention on the compelling idea that biased expectancies in a culture, more perhaps than any other variable, disrupt literacy and that his imbalance can only be corrected when these forces become recognized for their contribution to incidence of reading failure.

The effects of differences in sex role socialization were evident in many aspects of behavior and expectations in boys and girls. One area of profound meaning for society in general and individuals in particular is the effect such differences between the sexes assert in occupational preferences and achievement in school. Approaching this topic from different perspectives Cathleen Brown in the United States and Corinne Hutt in England studied vocational choice in boys and girls. Dr. Brown found that girls in high school persisted in their stereotypic expectations of careers. She attributed this persistence, in spite of recent legislation and social movements, to the fact that such beliefs are nonconscious. She advocates for school programs which permit discussion of the issues involved in choosing an occupation. It is her belief that decisions which are based on conscious choice are effective for eliminating stereotypes.

Dr. Hutt stresses the asymmetry between feminine and masculine roles deriving from several distinct sources. She states that the current emphasis on equal achievement and hence competition between boys and girls ignores differences in aptitudes between the sexes and may place an entirely unwarranted expectation for accomplishment on girls. The use of this interpretation of dissonance between ability and aspiration ignores some of the recent criticisms regarding the errors in this traditional explanation of differential achievement. In the United States, where mixed sex schools are more generally the rule, this older explanation has begun to dissipate as girls entry into courses of study considered "more challenging", i.e., male dominated, tends to increase. More fundamentally achievement difference studies have ignored the self-fulfilling aspect of differences in expectation and the weight of stereotypic influences on thinking and behaving. It certainly must be acknowledged that in the furor over sex role socialization we run the risk of reducing the complexity of development to over simplification of processes and issues.

One encouraging contribution for reducing potential competition along gender lines is that of cross-sex friendship in the elementary schools. Adma d'Heurle and her colleagues reported on a study preliminary to direct assessment of cross-sex friendship. To prepare the ground for this study they reviewed the content of readers available to school children in Sweden and the United States. Just as Abu Nasr in Lebanon found texts to be a potential source for inducing change in attitudes about sex roles, so too, does d'Huerle consider this in preparing her study. The differences in readers between the two cultures, with respect to friendships, appeared to be negligible. In Swedish texts there was more evidence of presenting social problems of serious consequence. Both sets of texts seemed to deal more with male friendship. American texts emphasized winning and achievement as prominent themes, while Swedish texts presented an image of children as more dependent upon the guidance and direction of adults. In a corollary sociometric questionnaire children from both countries declared their preference for the same sex in doing homework together and in sharing a secret. Boys tended slightly more than girls to make cross-sex choices in these two tasks. Once again this difference can be accounted for in the same way that other participants such as Leung, Hutt, and Brown argue. Basically, the preferential treatment of boys seems to encourage more sharply defined limits of acceptable behavior. Perhaps it is the clarity of role dimensions, as well as a greater sense of security, that combine to permit boys to explore behaviors beyond those limits. Several of the studies reported at these workshops have confirmed that socialization tends to cleave to the ideological lines of a culture. The observed bifurcation of sex stereotyping is not a universal imperative linked to a particular requirement or stage of development. It is rather more or less a reflection of the trends and emphases fostered in a particular culture.

Most of the studies reported in the workshops describe children in school and only one dealt with concerns from a broader ethological standpoint. Charles Downing considers the reasons boys experience more road accidents than girls. The facts are unequivocal with regard to the number of accidents between the sexes. Boys sustain nearly twice as many pedestrian and pedal vehicle accidents than girls. Other studies have offered the view that stereotyped male characteristics, aggression in particular, are related to vulnerability to traffic accidents. Downing has avoided any attempt to reduce the complexities of his observations to simplifications regarding the underlying nature of the relationship between prevalence and behavior. He states that his study, like so many others, does not shed light on the presumed origins of these relationships. He considers the attempt to distinguish innate characteristics from those which may be culturally induced as an essentially insoluble problem.

Surely, as has been observed so often, the tendency to pit one against the other in topics which involve biological and cultural variables is, indeed, a problem without solution. At a more fundamental level this misconstrues the respective contributions of innate tendencies and cultural shaping to individual behavior. In an era during which sociobiology, ethology, and the social sciences in general have been both unwittingly and intentionally drawn into ideological battles, it would appear that more caution should be observed than the facile extrapolations from very tentative evidence for support of extreme positions. Are the sexes innately different, and in what significant ways? These questions still beg for answers. At this juncture we need more powerful theoretical contributions than has been the case to date. Certainly the scientific quest for knowledge, which should motivate such arguments, cannot languish in the background to be overshadowed by the polemics of social movements. Such a consequence serves no useful end and makes a mockery of the desire to correct obvious social shortcomings. What emerges a modern social alchemy whose touchstone is derision rather than sound arguments supported by a valid body of empirical evidence.

The papers in the two workshops have labored under the shortcomings of extant knowledge and theory. Often the presenters have decried the limits imposed by the state of knowledge and have managed with the conceptual and methodological tools available to contribute significantly to advancing our understanding through refinement in arguments, clarification of concepts, distinctions in terminology, and, above all, to test empirically the complicated questions they pose. A summary cannot do justice to the intricacies of argumentation and implication broached in these workshops. Our examination of the current state of affairs in sex role socialization must analyze relevant issues in a spirit of respect for the complexity of personal and social reasons for the existence of such arrangements. So far the changes in traditional arrangements have been negligible compared to the change which seems imminent. The change appears imminent because the larger structure in which our central sexual arrangements is embedded — human societal life as a whole — has reached a crucial phase in its own development.[2]

A human social (or interpersonal psychological) system, unlike any other biological system can strive to become conscious of its own processes of growth and self maintenance ... the only kind, so far as we know, in which it is possible for living order to be envisioned beforehand and then arrived at voluntarily from within.[3]

In summary then, we must recognize that

Without that central feature of our symbiotic gender arrangements — central because it bears on the ultimate meaning of our life, the ultimate character of our place in the order of things, and (b) because it is the coordinating matrix for all the other features, the kingpin that has held them together, the fulcrum around which the tensions they generate have been balanced — the rest of the arrangement crumbles. On the other hand there is in the dying old arrangement that which we all have to outgrow or die ourselves; and on the other hand what there is in it that we all legitimately need, that we cannot and should not try to do without, and that we must therefore find other ways of getting.[4,5]

University of Rhode Island

NOTES

*   Thanks are due to Dr Susan Bram who contributed her thoughts, comments and editorial ideas to this Introduction.

1 Leung's paper, entitled 'Sex Roles of Children in the People's Republic of China', is not included in this volume.
2 Dinnerstein, D., *The Mermaid and the Minotaur: Sexual Arrangements and Human Malaise*, Harper and Row/Colophon, New York, 1977, p. 252.
3 Ibid., p. 256.
4 Ibid., p. 277.
5 Special appreciation is expressed to Adma d'Heurle for her assistance in preparing this Introduction and her selection of the quotations from Dinnerstein.

FELICISIMA C. SERAFICA, Ph.D. and SUZANNA ROSE, Ph.D.

PARENTS' SEX ROLE ATTITUDES AND CHILDREN'S CONCEPTS OF FEMININITY AND MASCULINITY*

The title of the workshop to which this paper is presented asks whether parents', teachers', and children's attitudes toward sex roles are changing. Most likely, the organizers of this symposium were moved to ask this question because of the secular changes taking place in the countries represented at this conference. The fact that this issue of changing sex role attitudes is being raised implies that such changes may have important psychological implications. From a developmental-clinical perspective, the most obvious implication of such a question is that changes in parents', teachers', and children's sex role attitudes may result in altered socialization patterns. In this paper, we will briefly review the available evidence regarding changes in sex role standards and attitudes, then discuss the development of children's concepts of masculinity and femininity, and how this might be influenced by parents' sex role attitudes and children's friendship choices. Finally, the implications of changes in parents' and peers' sex role attitudes on the developing child's concepts of masculinity and femininity will be explored. Our general aims are: (1) to delineate some conceptual and method-ological issues in the study of how sex role concepts evolve, and (2) to suggest some directions for future research. It seems appropriate, prior to reviewing the psychological research literature on changes in sex role attitudes, to define one's terms. In this paper, a distinction is made between the terms "sex role standards" and "sex role attitudes." The former is used in referring to the societal norms regarding appropriate characteristics and behaviors for men and for women. In contrast, the latter term is employed to mean a person's point of view or feeling about a given set of sex role standards. Thus, sex role standards refer to a society's belief system about the distinctions between men and women whereas sex role attitudes refer to whether or not an individual considers those beliefs valid, as well as the degree of flexibility associated with the implementation of such beliefs. Both terms may be further differentiated from "sex role preference" which refers to the extent to which an individual accepts, values, and incorporates those behaviors and characteristics society considers appropriate for his/her gender. Sex role attitudes and sex role preference are predicated on an awareness of sex role standards. The term "sex role concepts" is used here to refer to an individual's knowledge about sex role standards or norms for men (concept of masculinity) and women (concept of femininity).

CHANGING SEX ROLES?

Given the recent attention to the limitations rigid adherence to traditional sex role imposes on children and adults, it is quite often assumed that sex role

11

I. Gross, J. Downing, and A. d'Heurle (eds.), Sex Role Attitudes and Cultural Change, 11–24.
Copyright © 1982 by D. Reidel Publishing Company.

standards, attitudes and preferences are in a state of flux. Challenges issued largely by the feminist movement have argued strongly that gender *not* be used as the criterion for determining which characteristics and behaviors are "appropriate" for boys and girls. Claiming that traditional masculinity and femininity are psychologically and behaviorally confining, some researchers, such as Sandra Bem, are now attempting to empirically support their position. In fact, Bem (1975) was able to demonstrate that highly "masculine" men and "feminine" women were less willing to engage in opposite sex-role behaviors, e.g., cooking and carpentry activity, respectively, than were less sex-typed males and females.

There is not much evidence, however, to support the assumption that this controversy has resulted in changes in sex role standards. A 1972 study by Broverman, et al., of adults' (17–60 years) sex role stereotypes did not differ greatly from a 1957 investigation of college students by Sherriffs and McKee. In both, males and females regarded men as significantly more "aggressive," "independent," "unemotional," and "logical" than women; whereas women were described as significantly more "gentle," "tactful," and "tender" than men. Furthermore, Der-Karabetian and Smith (1977) found that high school and college students were still using these same traditional ways of describing men and women. Hence, it seems reasonable to conclude that sex role standards have not changed much over the past 20 years.

CHANGES IN SEX ROLE ATTITUDES

There is somewhat more support for the conclusion that sex role *attitudes* are changing. For instance, Broverman et al. (1972) reported that subjects were more likely to rate masculine traits as socially desirable. However, in the Der-Karabetian and Smith (1977) investigation, males did not differentially value masculine and feminine characteristics, and females valued feminine characteristics *more* than masculine traits — in direct contrast to the Broverman et al. findings.

Changes in sex role attitudes were also reported by Ruble, Croke, Frieze and Parsons (1975) in two field studies using college women. Women's studies students were found to become less traditional in their attitudes from the pre- to the post-test relative to the students in the comparison (developmental psychology) classes. Significant attitude change occurred in beliefs concerning traditional roles of women, stereotypes regarding the natural capacities and vocations of men and women, and perception of sex discrimination, but not with respect to personal expectations concerning a career and a family, and distrust and dislike of women.

Similar results were found by Porter (Gump, 1972) in an investigation of the sex role attitudes of female junior and senior college students. As reported by Gump (1972), the view of femininity most acceptable to the subjects was one which attested to the importance and feasibility of assuming the roles of wife and mother, while concomitantly pursuing careers. However, since many of the women in the study were planning to have families and most were pursuing careers traditional for women, Gump concluded that the subjects were not proposing radical alternatives to the traditional view.

Thus, it *does* appear that sex role attitudes may be undergoing some change. Nevertheless, as indicated by the Ruble et al. (1975) and Gump (1972) studies, attitude change was not accompanied by a concomitant change in personal sex role preferences. Most of the women were still in agreement with the marriage and motherhood aspects of the traditional female role, preferring it for themselves. The effect of changing sex role attitudes on males' sex role preferences, however, has not been established.

In summary, based on these reports, recent secular trends have not made a significant impact on sex role standards and preferences. Although it is possible that traditional sex role differentiations are breaking down, most of the changes seem to be affecting attitudes rather than preferences or standards. Even so, changes in the belief systems are occurring slowly and are primarily in response to specific conditions such as taking a women's studies course (Ruble et al., 1975). Furthermore, certain sex role beliefs are more amenable to change than others. As Emmerich (1973) has noted, "secular changes in sex roles are not all of one piece; they selectively influence different aspects of sex role behavior and do so differentially among subpopulations." (p. 125)

CONCEPTS OF MASCULINITY AND FEMININITY

The multifaceted nature of sex role development is now generally acknowledged by scientific investigators with differing theoretical orientations. A complete account of sex role development must include: (1) the developmental sequence for each aspect, (2) the relationships between the various aspects at different levels of development, and (3) the variables which influence developmental trends and the mechanisms involved. The focus of this paper is on concepts of masculinity and femininity, i.e., sex role concepts. These concepts reflect the individual's knowledge and understanding about the sex role standard which prevail in his/her particular society. It is our contention that these concepts involve more than just a memory bank consisting of information about sex role standards learned by a person in the course of growing up. Rather they are organized conceptual systems whose forms change as a function of cognitive development.

Among theories of sex role development, Kohlberg's (1966) cognitive-developmental formulation seems most useful as a basis for understanding the evolution of sex role concepts. Kohlberg (1966) has proposed that sex role development occurs in the following sequence. First, the young child becomes aware that humans come in two sexes and that he/she falls into one of these groups. Out of this awareness emerges the child's gender identity, i.e., cognitive categorization of self as "boy" or "girl." Kohlberg suggests further that this judgment, based on a physical reality, is made early in the child's life and acquires greater constancy with increasing age. Studies conducted by DeVries (1969, 1974) and Thompson (1975) have yielded some support for Kohlberg's hypotheses about the emergence of gender identity and the child's understanding of gender constancy.

Secondly, following the establishment of gender identity, the child begins to categorize objects and events in the physical and social environment on the basis of sex. The products of this categorization process involving gender identity as the organizing principle are the child's concepts of masculinity and femininity, i.e., sex role concepts. According to Kohlberg (1966), the attributes of sex role concepts become value-laden. There is an inherent tendency in the child to value same-sex characteristics, behaviors, etc., a propensity which serves the function of maintaining cognitive consistency for him/her. As a result of this different valuing, the child also begins to imitate sex-appropriate behaviors and to avoid sex-inappropriate behaviors and objects. Also during this period, the child starts to model the behaviors of same-sex individuals, particularly those of the same-sex parent.

Finally, after differential values are established and the rudiments of sex role concepts and sex-appropriate behaviors are acquired, identification with same-sex figures, in particular the same-sex parent occurs. Kohlberg (1966) posits that the desire to be masculine or feminine instills a wish to imitiate a masculine or feminine model as the case may be, which, in turn, strengthens the emotional attachment to the model.

It is our view that in contrast to the development of cognition as conceptualized by Piaget (1947) and of moral judgment as formulated earlier by Piaget (1932), then by Kohlberg (1963), the sequence for sex role development described above is not a structural sequence representing changes in form. Rather, Kohlberg appears to be describing three important aspects of sex role development which are interrelated but have different points of onset and are characterized by different developmental trends. As indicated earlier, our primary interest in this paper is in the second aspect, sex role concepts.

Kohlberg (1966) has not provided us with an explicit account of the sequence in which concepts of masculinity or femininity are evolved in the maturing child. On the basis of findings from studies of person perception in children (Livesley & Bromley, 1973; Scarlett, Press, & Crockett, 1971; Peevers & Secord, 1973), it is hypothesized that children's concepts of masculinity and femininity are initially global or relatively undifferentiated; with increasing age, greater differentiation and hierarchic integration takes place. Thus, some attributes come to be considered as more fundamental and critical than others. Furthermore, the earliest attributes comprising this category system are concrete, e.g., clothing and hair (Conn, 1940; Conn and Kanner, 1947; Katcher, 1955; Thompson & Bentler, 1971), with psychological qualities being added later on. Corollary to the development of sex role concepts, there are changes taking place in the attitudes about sex role standards. Initially, maleness or femaleness have neutral value. Gradually, maleness and femaleness become polarized. Sex role norms consistent with the child's gender identity are positively valued (Kohlberg, 1966) and maintained through reinforcement provided by the parents and other significant adults in the child's environment (Mischel, 1970). Through the latter, the child also learns that people attach positive or negative value to role prescriptions. Hence, a rejection of the opposite pole may occur, in varying degrees among different children. This has been found, particularly in young boys who show an active dislike for and denigration of females and female-linked behaviors, characteristics and objects (e.g., Hartup, Moore, & Sager, 1963; Lynn, 1964). This polarized attitude about sex roles is not confined to young children. It can continue well into adulthood (Rebecca, Hefner, & Oleshansky, 1972; Hefner, Rebecca, & Oleshansky, 1975). In children, it is unavoidable because of the difficulty they have in focusing on and in coordinating multiple perspectives (Piaget, 1966; Selman & Byrne, 1973; Shantz, 1975) as well as reconciling apparent contradictions in feelings and attitudes (Harter, 1977). With increasing cognitive maturity, the child comes to realize that masculinity-femininity judgements usually involve more than one dimension. Furthermore, there is increasing recognition that sex role standards are not imperative nor absolute, that they are associated with sociocultural and historical conditions, applied relatively depending upon the specific situation. Thus, a more flexible attitude about sex role standards and their implementation emerges. The distinguishing characteristic of such an attitude is its flexibility; individuals with this kind of attitude would exhibit male-type or female-type behaviors in accordance with situational demands. Our account of developmental changes in sex role attitudes is very similar to the description given by Hefner et al. (1975) of sex role development. We prefer, however, to postulate the sequence only for sex role attitudes and posit that, in ontogenesis, the logical necessity for the sequence is implied by the developmental changes taking place in the individual's cognitive structures.

Fundamental aims for a developmental analysis of sex role concepts include establishing the onset of the masculine-feminine categorizing process (more commonly referred to as sex-typing), determining whether the evolution of sex role concepts and attitudes follows the respective sequences postulated for them, describing in greater detail the content and form of thought at various levels, and examining the relationships between independent variables and developmental trends.

The onset of sex typing has received a great deal of attention from scientific investigators. It is now known that as early as 24 months of age, infants can sort stereotyped articles methodically in response to instructions to put things for mothers and girls in one box and things for fathers and boys in another box; this ability improves with age such that 30- and 36-month-olds are significantly better at the task than the 24-month-olds (Thompson, 1975). In studies using either a sorting technique or requiring subjects to attribute toy preferences to the IT figure, it has been consistently found that by 4 to 6 years of age, most children are able to discriminate between items socially prescribed for females and those for males (Brown, 1956; Nadelman, 1974; Schell & Silber, 1968; Thompson, 1975; Thompson & Bentler, 1973).

Much less is known about the sex role concepts of older children, adolescents, and adults. The few studies available suggest that sex role concepts don't change very much past the age of seven. Hartley & Hardesty (1964) did not find age to be reliably related to the ability of 5-, 8-, and 11-year-old children from a middle class background to indicate whether a boy or a girl would play in a certain setting or with a particular object and engage in a specific type of activity. Using a picture story technique, Williams, Bennett, & Best (1975) found a significant increase in knowledge of sex stereotypes from kindergarten to second grade but only in those subjects tested by male examiners. Moreover, there was no further increment by fourth grade. In a study involving a wider age range (seventh grade, twelfth grade, and adult) and using an Attitude Check List of traits considered desirable in a male or female target ideal, Urberg & Labouvie-Vief (1976), failed to find empirical support for their hypothesis that late adolescence and adult-hood would be characterized by a relative degree of sex role specialization. Instead, age related patterns mainly reflected an increased endorsement of sex role stereotypes.

The foregoing results may indeed reflect the true state of affairs. If so, Kohlberg's assumptions about the cognitive basis of sex role development would seem unfounded. These results are more consistent with a social learning perspective which posits that sex role standards are learned directly or indirectly, and maintained through differential reinforcement. However, perhaps the measures used in these studies were not sensitive enough to developmental changes in sex role concepts which occur in later years. Essentially, they were exemplars of a forced choice technique which may have masked the greater differentiation and hierarchic integration characterizing sex role concepts at higher levels of development. Also, as Urberg and Labouvie-Vief (1976) said of their measure, these were not designed to assess the ability to differentiate situation-specific aspects of sex role expectations. Furthermore, these results seem contrary to what would be expected concerning adults' sex role attitudes and preferences based on life span development studies. Two of these (Lowenthal, Thurnker, & Chirilboga, 1975; Maas & Juypers, 1974) found sex differences in attitudes and behaviors at one life stage that were reversed at a large stage, suggesting at least the possibility of related developmental changes in sex role concepts and attitudes. There is still a need, therefore, for a study assessing transformations in sex role concepts during the life span preferably using the clinical interview technique which has proven so useful in studies of children's concepts about various physical (Piaget, 1929, 1930, 1952) and social (Elkind, 1961, 1962, 1963; Piaget, 1932) phenomena. Such a method would yield information about what children at different ages take to be the critical attributes and correlates of sex role concepts and their notions about the constancy of the different attributes. In addition, as suggested earlier by Emmerich (1973), a developmental analysis of when and how the child's descriptive (what people do) and normative (what people ought to do) concepts become differentiated also seems indicated. According to Emmerich, this ability to distinguish descriptive and normative aspects of sex role may be a relatively late developmental achievement.

PARENTAL INFLUENCES ON CHILDREN'S SEX ROLE CONCEPTS

During a symposium on sex role identification held in the early sixties, Lynn (1964) commented that there is a paucity of research concerning specific sex-typing practices used by parents. Our survey of the psychological literature suggests that Lynn's (1964) statement is still an apt description of the state of the art in this field, in spite of the increased attention paid to sex role development in recent years. The majority of studies have attempted to relate parental characteristics and reported behaviors to the offspring's sex role preferences, perception of self as masculine or feminine, or sex-typed behavior (Biller, 1968; Hetherington, 1965, 1967; Levy, 1943; Meyers, 1944; Mussen & Distler, 1959; Mussen & Rutherford, 1963; Payne & Mussen, 1956). Mischel (1970) cautions that the relationships found in these studies are of modest magnitude, and generally have been difficult to replicate. He suggests paying more attention to the concrete contingencies employed by parents for reinforcing sex-typed behaviors and to the sex-typed patterns modeled by parents and peers.

There have been a few attempts to more directly assess specific parental reactions to children's sex-typed behavior. Fling and Manosevitz (1972) scored parental responses on a modified IT test and interview for differential reinforcement and modeling of sex-typed interests. The only significant correlation they found between parental measures and aspects of sex role development were between Encouragement, i.e., making available, teaching, suggesting, approving, participating in, and modeling sex appropriate interests, and Adoption, i.e., child's responses to what do you like to play with the most or a lot, scores of fathers and daughters, respectively. There was a similar trend ($p < .06$) for mothers' Encouragement and sons' Adoption scores.

Rothbart and Maccoby (1966) elicited parental reactions to a series of 12 verbal statements delivered in a child's gender-neutral voice that the parents were asked to imagine was the voice of their four-year-old child at home playing. Although a significant interaction between sex of parent and sex of child emerged in that both fathers and mothers were more permissive of aggressive and dependent behaviors from the opposite-sex child than from the same sex child, the results in general failed to confirm the hypothesis that parents' sex role stereotypes would be reflected in their reactions to the sex-typed behaviors of their children. This hypothesis was further investigated by Atkinson and Endsley (1976) among parents of four- to six-year-old children, using a questionnaire instead of audio-taped-recorded questions rendered in a child's voice. The authors of this study concluded that their results provide relatively clear support for the hypothesis that parents respond to their children's behavior in a way that reflects the parents' preference for and encouragement of stereotypic sex-role behaviors. Since there was no attempt in this study to independently assess the parents' knowledge of the prevailing sex role standards or their sex role preferences and attributes, this conclusion seems premature.

In order to demonstrate the relationship between parental variables (e.g., sex role concepts, sex role preferences) and child rearing practices or their outcomes, measures of the independent as well as the dependent variables should be included. Unfortunately, although there are well-established measures of sex role preferences and perceptions of self as masculine or feminine, very little work has been done so far in developing measures of parents' sex role concepts and attitudes, particularly in regards to children and adolescents at different ages. The availability of such measures, assuming that they meet psychometric standards, would permit us to search for answers to such questions as the degree of congruence between parental sex role concepts or attitudes and their child-rearing practices, and between parents' and children's sex role concepts or attitudes at different ages of the offspring. More importantly, for those of us who are interested in the impact of recent secular trends, the presence of such measures would allow us to assess changes in parents' sex role concepts or attitudes or to make comparisons between those who hold traditional versus contemporary views.

Assuming that the methodological problems are worked out successfully, there are a number of potentially fruitful avenues to explore concerning the parental behaviors which mediate the impact of their sex role concepts and attitudes on those of their offspring. Mussen (1969) described two clusters of parental behaviors which may be related to the development of sex role concepts. The first cluster, tuition, consists of such behaviors as verbal statements which directly impart and/or explain information pertaining to sex role standards, differential rewards and punishments, respectively, for sex-appropriate and sex-inappropriate responses, and other instructional or guiding activities. The second cluster is comprised of those ways through which the parent provides a model for the child to emulate. We submit that there is a third cluster of behaviors which for want of a better term will momentarily be referred to as "structuring the environment."

Parental efforts at structuring the child's environment which reflect their sex role concepts start even before the child is born in their choice of a name or the nursery decor or the color of the layette and other articles necessary for the infant. After birth, structuring the environment may take such forms as selective purchase of toys, clothes and other articles, arranging certain activities for the child as opposed to others, and encouraging certain friendship while ignoring or even discouraging others. The work of Hartley (1964) as well as Rheingold and Cook (1975) suggest that more attention should be paid by investigators of socialization practices to how parents structure the child's environment.

During the early years, just when children are beginning to acquire sex role concepts, they are very dependent upon their parents for peer interaction opportunities. Except when in nursery school (and this, too, is chosen by the parents), young children play mostly with peers whom their parents have invited over or whose parents invite them. Thus, a young child's initial friends are essentially chosen for him by his parents and may thereby reflect, from a sex role perspective, whom they regard as sex-appropriate friendship choices for their child.

PEER INFLUENCES ON SEX ROLE CONCEPTS

In late childhood, opportunities for peer interaction widen and parents have less influence over children's friendship choices. The child's circle of friends may include youngsters who have been exposed to a different set of sex role standards. Interaction with such peers is also likely to affect the development of sex role concepts. It has been also suggested by Brim (1958) and Rosenberg and Smith (1968) that the child's sex role learning is not based merely on the same sex parent but is also substantially influenced by other children. According to Hetherington (1967), sex role preferences (and by implication, sex role concepts) become increasingly influenced by social norms. When this occurs, the relationship between sex typing and parental behaviors may become attenuated.

Kohlberg's theoretical formulation of sex role development would predict that the young child would prefer friends of the same sex. There is ample support for this prediction. Sex of the child is a more important determinant of friendship choice than race (Asher, Oden, & Gottman, 1976). An early study by Criswell (1939) showed that the gap between the sexes was greater than racial cleavage and that classmates of the same sex but different race were nearly always preferred by a given group of boys or girls to those of the same race but different sex. This trend was also found in more recent studies by Asher (1973) and Singleton (1974). When cross-sex friendships are formed, they tend to be much less stable than same-sex friendships (Gronlund, 1955).

The propensity for same-sex friendships reflects the child's tendency to positively value sex-appropriate characteristics. This valuing is enhanced by the friends since they, too, share the value. Like parents, friends serve as models and provide differential rewards and punishments, respectively, for sex-appropriate and sex-inappropriate behaviors. They are also sources of new information leading to elaboration of the concept. Friends, in contrast to parents, are much more likely to interact with the child in a manner calculated to induce cognitive conflict resulting in restructuring of sex role concepts. First, friends may have had different experiences or been exposed to some differing viewpoints. Secondly, being immature themselves they are apt to be less cautious about introducing contradictory information and challenging the child's beliefs. Since children's friendships tend to be cross-age (Graziano, French, Brownell, & Hartup, 1976), exposure to divergent viewpoints is inevitable. Friendships, therefore, may play a more important role in the development of sex role concepts and attitudes in older children and adolescents. Whether or not sex role concepts and attitudes change may be more closely related to the influence of friends than of parents.

IMPLICATIONS OF SECULAR CHANGES

It is interesting to speculate on the effects of ongoing secular changes on parents' and peers' sex role concepts and attitudes and how such changes would affect development. Parents for whom flexibility in sex roles is a salient aspect of their childrearing efforts may actively choose environments for their child that is flexible on this dimension. That a growing number of parents are concerned with this is evident from the amount of recent literature on "nonsexist" education (Frazier & Sadker, 1973; Olsen, 1977; Scott, 1972). Conceivably, this environmental structuring may also involve parental preferences for cross-sex or "androgynous" playmates for their sons or daughters. Since peer influences on children's sex role concepts and attitudes are presumed to be fairly important, a nontraditional peer environment may influence the content or order of sex role learning. Pertinent research questions arising from this line of thinking focus on the nature of the link between parents' and children's sex role attitudes. If parents acquire a more flexible attitude, i.e., function at the stage of sex role transcendence posited by Rebecca et al. (1976), will a similar attitude also be exhibited by the young child? Is sex role conformity or nonconformity a determinant of parent preferences for their child's friends? And finally, will a child in a nontraditional peer group demonstrate a concomitant flexibility in sex role attitudes? That this might happen can be predicted from a social learning theory perspective. Cognitive developmental theorists would argue otherwise. From this latter perspective, the developmental sequence would remain the same; however the rate of change might be accelerated and performance would more often reflect competence. Cognitive developmental theory would also predict that the effects of changes in parents' and peers' sex role concepts on the developing child would vary at different ages. It is hoped that empirically-based answers to some of these issues will emerge at this workshop.

The Ohio State University (F.C.S.)
University of Missouri at St. Louis (S.R.)

NOTE

*　An earlier version of this paper was presented at a Workshop on 'Parents', Teachers' and Children's Attitudes toward Sex Roles − at Crossroads?', held during the 1977 World Congress on Mental Health, Vancouver, B. C., Canada, August, 1977.

REFERENCES

Asher, S. R.
　1973 The influence of race and sex on children's sociometric choices across the school
　　　year. Unpublished manuscript, University of Illinois.
Asher, S. R., Oden, S. L., & Gottman, J. M.
　In press Children's friendships in school settings. Quarterly Review of Early Education.
Atkinson, J., and Endsley, R. C.
　1976 Influence of sex of child and parent on parental reactions to hypothetical parent-
　　　child situations. Genetic Psychology Monographs 94: 131–147.
Bem, S. L.
　1975 Sex role adaptability – one consequence of psychological androgyny. Journal of
　　　Personality and Social Psychology 31: 634–643.
Biller, H. B.
　1968 A note on father absence and masculine development in lower-class Negro and
　　　white boys. Child Development 39: 1003–1006.
Brim, O. G.
　1958 Family structure and sex role learning by children: a further analysis of Helen
　　　Koch's data. Sociometry 21: 1–15.
Brown, D. G.
　1956 Sex role preference in young children. Psychological Monographs 70, No. 14.
Conn, J. H.
　1940 Children's reactions to the discovery of genital differences. American Journal of
　　　Orthopsychiatry 10: 747–755.
Conn, J. H., and Kanner, L.
　1947 Children's awareness of sex differences. Journal of Child Psychiatry 1: 3–57.
Criswell, J. H.
　1939 A sociometric study of race cleavage in the classroom. Archives of Psychology
　　　No. 235: 1–82.
Der-Karabetian, A., and Smith, A. J.
　1977 Sex role sterotyping in the US: is it changing? Sex Roles 3.
DeVries, R.
　1969 Constancy of generic identity in the years three to six. Monographs of the Society
　　　for Research in Child Development 34 (Whole No. 3, Serial No. 127).
DeVries, R.
　1974 Relationship among Piagetian, IQ, and achievement assessments. Child Develop-
　　　ment 45: 746–756.
Elkind, D.
　1961 The child's conception of his religious denomination: I. The Jewish child. Journal
　　　of Genetic Psychology 99: 209–225.
Elkind, D.
　1962 The child's conception of his religious denomination: II. The Catholic child.
　　　Journal of Genetic Psychology 101: 185–193.
Elkind, D.
　1963 The child's conception of his religious denomination: III. The Protestant child.
　　　Journal of Genetic Psychology 103: 291–304.
Emmerich, W.
　1973 Socialization and sex-role development. In P. B. Baltes and K. W. Schaie (eds.),
　　　Life-span developmental psychology: Personality and socialization. New York:
　　　Academic Press.
Fling, S., and Manosevitz, M.
　1972 Sex typing in nursery school children's play interests. Developmental Psychology
　　　7: 146–152.

Frazier, N., and Sadker, M.
   1973 Sexism in School and Society. New York: Harper and Row.
Graziano, W., French, D., Brownell, C. A., and Hartup, W. W.
   1976 Peer interaction in same- and mixed-age triads in relation to chronological age and incentive condition. Child Development 47: 707–714.
Gronlund, N. E.
   1959 Sociometry in the Classroom. New York: Harper.
Harter, S.
   1977 A cognitive-developmental approach to children's expression of conflicting feelings and a technique to facilitate such expression in play therapy. Journal of Consulting and Clinical Psychology 45: 417–432.
Hartley, R. E.
   1964 A developmental view of female sex role definition and identification. Merrill-Palmer Quarterly 10: 3–15.
Hartley, R. E., and Hardesty, F. P.
   1964 Children's perceptions of sex roles in childhood. Journal of Genetic Psychology 105: 45–51.
Hartup, W. W., Moore, S. G., and Sager, G.
   1963 Avoidance of inappropriate sex typing by young children. Journal of Consulting Psychology 27: 467–473.
Hefner, R., Rebecca, M., and Oleshansky, B.
   1975 Development of sex-role transcendence. Human Development 18: 143–158.
Hetherington, E. M.
   1967 The effects of familial variables on sex typing, on parent-child similarity, and on imitation in children. In J. P. Hill (ed.), Minnesota Symposium on Child Psychology, Vol. 1: 82–107.
Katcher, A.
   1955 The discrimination of sex differences by young children. Journal of Genetic Psychology 87: 131–143.
Kohlberg, L.
   1963 The development of children's orientations toward a moral order. Vita Humana 6: 11–33.
Kohlberg, L.
   1966 A cognitive-developmental analysis of children's sex role concepts and attitudes. In E. E. Maccoby (ed.), The Development of Sex Differences. Stanford, California: Stanford University Press.
Levy, D. M.
   1943 Maternal overprotection. New York: Columbia University Press.
Lynn, D. B.
   1964 Divergent feedback and sex role identification in boys and men. Merrill-Palmer Quarterly 10: 17–23.
Livesley, W. J., and Bromley, D. B.
   1973 Person Perception in Childhood and Adolescence. London: Wiley.
Lowenthal, M. F., Thurnher, M., Chiriboga, D., and Associate
   1975 Four Stages of Life. Washington: Jossey-Bass.
Maas, H. S., and Kuypers, J. A.
   1974 From Thirty to Seventy: A Longitudinal Study of Adult Lifestyles and Personality. San Francisco: Jossey-Bass.
Meyers, C. E.
   1944 The effect of conflicting authority on the child. University of Iowa Studies in Child Welfare 20, No. 409: 31–98.

Mischel, W.
  1970 Sex-typing and socialization. In P. H. Mussen (ed.), Carmichael's Manual of Child Psychology. New York: Wiley.
Mussen, P. H.
  1969 Early sex role development. In D. A. Goslin (ed.), Handbook of Socialization Theory and Research. Chicago: Rand McNally, 708–731.
Mussen, P., and Distler, L.
  1959 Masculinity, identification and father-son relationships. Journal of Abnormal and Social Psychology 59: 350–356.
Mussen, P., and Rutherford, E.
  1963 Parent-child relations and parental personality in relation to young children's sex-role preferences. Child Development 34: 489–607.
Nadelman, L.
  1974 Sex identity in American children: memory, knowledge and preference tests. Developmental Psychology 10: 413–417.
Olsen, L.
  1977 Nonsexist Curricular Materials for Elementary Schools. Old Westbury, New York: The Feminist Press.
Payne, D. E., and Mussen, P. H.
  1956 Parent-child relations and father identification among adolescent boys. Journal of Abnormal and Social Psychology 52: 358–362.
Peevers, B. H., and Secord, P. F.
  1973 Developmental changes in attribution of descriptive concepts to persons. Journal of Personality and Social Psychology 27: 120–128.
Piaget, J.
  1929 The Child's Conception of the World. New York: Harcourt, Brace.
Piaget, J.
  1930 The Child's Conception of Physical Causality. London: Kegan Paul.
Piaget, J.
  1932 The Moral Judgment of the Child. Glencoe, Illinois: Free Press.
Piaget, J.
  1947 The Psychology of Intelligence. London: Routledge, Kegan Paul.
Piaget, J.
  1952 The Child's Conception of Number. New York: Humanities.
Piaget, J.
  1966 The Language and Thought of the Child. New York: Meridian.
Rebecca, M., Hefner, R., and Oleshansky, B.
  1976 A moderl of sex-role transcendence. Journal of Social Issues 32: 197–206.
Rheingold, H. L., and Cook, K. V.
  1975 The contents of boys' and girls' rooms as an index of parents' behaviors. Child Development 46: 459–464.
Rosenberg, B. G., and Sutton-Smith, B.
  1964 The measurement of masculinity and femininity in children: an extension and revalidation. Journal of Genetic Psychology 104: 259–264.
Rothbart, M. K., and Maccoby, E. E.
  1966 Parent's differential reactions to sons and daughters. Journal of Personality and Social Psychology 4: 237–243.
Shantz, C. U.
  1975 The development of social cognition. In E. M. Hetherington (ed.), Child Development Research, Vol. 5. Chicago: University of Chicago Press, 257–323.
Scott, A.
  1972 It's time for equal education. Ms, Oct.: 122–125.

Scarlett, H. H., Press, A. N., and Crockett, W. H.
   1971 Children's descriptions of peers: A Wernerian developmental analysis. Child
         Development 42: 439–455.
Schell, R. E. and Silber, J. W.
   1968 Sex-role discrimination among young children. Perceptual and Motor Skills 27:
         379–389.
Selman, R. L., and Byrne, D. F.
   1974 A structural-developmental analysis of levels of role-taking in middle childhood.
         Child Development 45: 803–807.
Sherriffs, A. C., and McKee, J. P.
   1957 Qualitative beliefs about men and women. Journal of Personality and Social
         Psychology 25: 451–464.
Singleton, L.
   1974 The effects of sex and race on children's sociometric choices for play and work.
         Urbana, Illinois: University of Illinois. (ERIC Document Reproduction Service
         No. ED 100 520)
Thompson, S. K., and Bentler, P. M.
   1971 The priority of cues in sex discrimination by children and adults. Developmental
         Psychology 5: 181–185.
Urberg, K. A., and Labouvie-Vief, G.
   1976 Conceptualizations of sex roles: A life-span developmental study. Developmental
         Psychology 12: 15–23.
Williams, J. E., Bennett, S. M., and Best, D. L.
   1975 Awareness and expression of sex stereotypes in young children. Developmental
         Psychology 11: 635–642.

MERRILL SARTY, Ph.D. and MAXENE JOHNSTON, R.N., M.A.

ETHNIC DIFFERENCES IN SEX STEREOTYPING BY MOTHERS: IMPLICATIONS FOR HEALTH CARE

ETHNOMEDICINE: STUDYING THE ROLE OF CULTURE IN HEALTH CARE

Health practitioners are becoming increasingly aware of the importance of the role of the social sciences in applied research. Traditional studies of health and human behavior, particularly when they are conducted among non-Western groups that are relatively uninfluenced by biomedical approaches, focus on alternatives to the usual biomedical meanings and implications of disease, illness, and health care. Such studies base their definitions on a community's own beliefs about illness and health-related practices. The underlying philosophy and techniques of anthropology consider the people being studied to be the specialists in whatever behavior is chosen for observation. In psychiatry (by contrast), it is the professional who is considered the expert specialist (Fabrega and Silver, 1973: 5). It might be said that in much of American psychology it too often appears that proof of a theoretical "concept" is the goal, and neither the observer nor the observed is of much intrinsic interest.

For the cultural anthropologist the set of categories, rules, and plans that cultures provide for their members, as a means of explaining and coping with life events, are not only highly patterned but also embedded in fundamental premises about the nature of reality and social relations (Fabrega and Silver, 1973: 223). As Mitchell has very recently pointed out, each society has its own right and wrong ways of doing things, from sharpening a pencil or an arrow to making love. There are also right and wrong ways of thinking. So it is that ideas, values, and notions about cause and effect are all learned products of one's culture. Because human beings are rarely neutral about any important aspect of their existence, behavior and values are usually permeated with, and circumscribed by, strong ethical constraints. The human predilection to institutionalize the many varied and sometimes conflicting approaches to living vividly separates us from other primates and may well provide the health practitioner materials for study and reflection (Mitchell, 1977: 16).

Unfortunately, we are all too often ethnocentric. Should we not instead be "ethnic centered"? By this term we mean to indicate not only our recognition that the patient is the center of our concerns, but also to imply that the patient is a product of his culture — a culture with tenets which we must accept and value as the equal of our own. As changes in contemporary society bring us closer to the image of the "melting pot", we find ourselves being propelled into proximity with those whose backgrounds and world views are far different from our own. Yet, ethnocentric upbringing and education often restrict our insight

25

I. Gross, J. Downing, and A. d'Heurle (eds.), Sex Role Attitudes and Cultural Change, 25–37.

into our own culturally-based ideas and values. Of course, such ethnocentricism can lead to an exaggeration and intensification of those elements of one's own folk-ways that are peculiar and that differentiate one group from others. While there may be positive effects of such an increasing ethnic identification, it can also lead to making value judgements and perceiving others not only as deviant, but wrong (LeVine and Campbell, 1972: 8). Western health practitioners. for instance, presume that independence and responsibility are important if not essential for any patient in a rehabilitation program, rarely realizing that these are culturally learned values and that not all patients share them (Torrey, 1972: 23).

It appears appropriate, therefore, that we should strive towards an approach that is not ethnocentric, but ethnic-centered. To this end, an understanding of cross-cultural beliefs, values and practices is essential.

Relevance of Cultural Patterns to Health Professionals

Such an understanding of ethnic differences has obvious relevance to health professionals. Two decades ago Margaret Mead suggested that patients from some cultures are apt to preserve their self-control better if they see as little of their relatives as possible; whereas patients from cultures with a different family structure will become depressed unless they are surrounded by a close, warm group of relatives (Mead, 1956: 260). Of course, whatever can be said of attitudes toward relatives can be said of a host of other attitudes bearing on health in general.

It also follows that mothers' perceptions concerning their children will be influenced by culture. Differences based on age and sex may be more or less extreme in different societies. Social behavior is certainly influenced by such other factors as kinship network, residence patterns, and the rules of that culture's role assignment and expectations (Whiting and Whiting, 1975: 59).

We hope that the process of successful parenting practices relating to health care will both benefit from an increased understanding of beliefs and value systems that parents hold concerning their children. Despite a considerable body of general knowledge, there is too little known about the issue of parental beliefs and values as they relate specifically to health and illness.

CULTURAL VARIATIONS IN SEX STEREOTYPING

One compelling issue in parenting has to do with the influence that sex stereo-typing may have on health-related attitudes and behavior.

Trends in General Society

The issue of sex stereotyping has come into focus in recent years, perhaps as a result of the women's movement specifically, and certainly as a function of increasing concerns with human rights in general. This interest in sex stereotyping has stimulated a critical examination of the concepts of masculinity and feminity and the cultural influences on the development of such concepts. Male and female stereotypes have been defined as the constellation of psychological traits generally attributed to men and women respectively. Thus, men are thought to be aggressive, forthright, strong, silent, and rational; while women are described as passive, indirect, weak, talkative, and emotional (Williams and Bennett, 1975: 327).

Sex stereotyping in a cross-cultural perspective has been examined recently by Georgene Seward (1977). She noted that, despite the promises of the Soviet revolution, sexist attitudes have not disappeared in Russia. Nor have the women freed themselves from deep-rooted occupational traditions. Despite the fact that women are nominally exempt from only two job categories (the "military underground", and command of small fishing boats) a recent survey of urban high school seniors showed a characteristic separation of vocational interests. Boys still prefer engineering, while girls are drawn to education and cultural pursuits. She cites studies concluding that the conflict and confusion so characteristic of women's attitudes contribute to a soaring divorce rate, and the scuttling of the Utopian dream of the early Soviet idealistis.

Sweden, on the other hand, because it avoided Russia's convulsive political upheavals and involvement in war, may offer a clearer picture of possibilities within a socialist state. Swedish attitudes have allowed a progressive, egalitarian social order in which liberalized laws govern marriage and divorce, and in which family planning is crucial. Their basic tenet is that sex differences concern only reproductive functions. Absolute emancipation of women and total equality of the sexes is assumed because there is no justification for putting people into the straightjackets of separate and distinct social roles. Freedom in the form of expanded options for women has brought with it a concomitant emancipation of men. So today there is the option to be a "househusband". However, small family size and residence patterns may also explain such distinctions.

Family Size and Sex Stereotypes

In another review of cross-cultural practices, Barry and his colleagues surveyed the process of socialization in 110 cultures. Most gave very different training to girls than they did to boys. There was a widespread pattern of greater pressure toward nurturance, obedience and responsibility in girls and toward self-reliance, achievement and striving in boys. From this study the authors inferred that the differences in socialization between the sexes in our society are no arbitrary custom of our culture, but rather an adaptive strategy to the "biological substratum of human life" (Barry, Bacon and Child, 1957: 329). Societies that emphasize differences in sex roles tend to have an economy that depends on superior strength and superior development of motor skills. It is interesting to note that such societies also have large families with close interaction. The implication for Western culture's nuclear family organization, is that sex differentiation cannot afford to be too great. To the extent that the nuclear family must stand alone, the man must be prepared to take the woman's role and vice-versa, when the partner is incapacitated or not present (Barry, Bacon and Child, 1957: 331).

Whether the Utopian ideal is being achieved in actuality, even in Sweden, is still open to debate. For many observers, it provides a most hopeful and socially adaptive model. There is a question, however, as to whether the current push for a "unisex" upbringing may not also cause problems. Whatever the ultimate adaptive value, our children may be getting an inappropriate preparation for an adult world that may remain sexist.

As much as we may hope for the realization of non-sexist attitudes in preparing children for changing adult roles it will be delayed so long as parents hold disparate sets of expectations for their boys and for their girls.

Throughout history sex-stereotyping has been transmitted by a process we call "cultural coding". Little boys (even as tiny infants) continue to be the objects of a father's exuberant roughhousing typically denied to little girls.

Children's toys are a revealing artifact of Western culture's approach to sex roles. In a recent study of sex-stereotyping in choice of toys for six-year-olds in upper-income American homes boys had a much greater variety of playthings than girls. Asked what they played with most often, girls named domestic toys and dolls while boys chose things designed for use outside the home, as they have done traditionally.

Sex Differences in the Incidence of Health Problems

After studying problem behavior of adolescents in the United States, Douvan found that males report a significantly higher frequency of aggression and feelings of resentment towards others, while females report a significantly higher frequency of feelings of tension and of psychosomatic symptoms. She concluded that disruptive behaviors precipitating adult intervention may be more characteristic of males because they are congruent with stereotypes of masculinity and are expressive of autonomy. Girls are believed to express stress in ways which do not precipitate adult intervention because aggressive behavior and challenging authority are incongruent with "femininity" (Douvan, 1977).

When one looks specifically at the realities of many of the current health problems of children, sex differentiation is often poignantly obvious. In both young children and adolescents the male to female ratio of suicides is approximately 3 to 1 (Rudolph, 1977: 837). The syndrome of sudden infant death strikes males over females by 3 to 2 (Rudolph, 1977: 832). Deaths due to drownings are almost 80 percent male. Schizophrenia and so-called "minimal brain dysfunction" are also reported more often in males. The work of Mechanic (1964) supports the idea that age is also an important factor in determining attitudes towards health risks. In his study of children, boys were found to be more stoic than girls, but older children were more stoic than younger children. These results are consistent with several other observations such as the higher utilization of medical facilities by women as compared with men, and the higher rate of accidents among boys, compared with girls of the same age (Anderson, 1963; Mellinger, 1963; Meyer, 1963).

Assumptions of Practitioner and Parent

Sex-stereotyping directly influences the value systems not only of parents but of the practitioner as well. Consider how practitioners prepare children for painful procedures in health settings. Do they not frequently encourage boys to be brave while handing girls tissues and encouraging their tears?

The work of Linda Fidell (1974) makes very clear the stereotypes presented to physicians in their medical journals. In an analysis of drug company advertising she noted that patients who were pictured with "real" physical complaints were most often men, while those with an expression of free-floating anxiety, low-back pain or insubstantial malaise requiring Valium were almost invariably women.

The drug companies, being astute merchandisers, may be leading the physician, but they may as likely be capitalizing on a ready-made situation. Women do make more than their share of visits to doctors. Though they bring fewer than their share of sky-divers' broken bones, they are more willing to present the subtle symptoms most readily diagnosed as "anxiety". Why should this be? Apart from the females having learned to be more dependent than the male (after all, she's more likely to ask directions when lost), she may be fulfilling a prophesy – a predictive message made clear by her mother's expectations.

Sex Stereotypes Affecting Health Decisions

Sex stereotuping related to health starts early in life. For example, in many parts of India, one ancient Hindu rite still observed is "annaprasan" or the rice-feeding ceremony. It is thought that the original purpose of this custom was to celebrate the baby's having survived the dangerous first half-year of life, but it also marks an important dietary milestone: the introduction of solid food. It is notable, however, that the ceremony is performed at six months of age for boys, but not until seven months for girls (Jelliffe, 1956: 670).

A California study of mothers' belief in the efficacy of vitamins noted very distinct sex stereotyping by mothers of small children. The subjects were equally divided among Anglos (Caucasians), English-speaking Mexican Americans (EMA), Spanish-speaking Mexican Americans (SMA), and Blacks living in Los Angeles. Questionnaires were supplemented with interviews. Results indicate that a mother's belief in vitamin efficacy is related to the sex of her child, and suggest that attitudes towards vitamins reflect ideas about medicine that are rooted in each ethnic group's respective folk culture. It is of interest that, in instances wherein mothers expressed greater "nonscientific" expectations, (expectations to which we applied the term "magical"), interactions with ethnicity occurred only with reference to data from mothers of girls. If those data will allow a couple of sweeping generalizations: it appeared that the Anglos and English-speaking Mexican American mothers of girls form a relatively homogeneous group (the ingroup?) contrasted with the Spanish-speaking Mexican Americans and Blacks (the outgroup?) Of these groups, the Anglos tended to distinguish least on the basis of sex, while the Spanish-speaking Mexican Americans made the strongest sex-based distinctions (Johnston and Sarty, 1975).

We are now in the process of analyzing data from a broader investigation of 240 mothers' attitudes and beliefs relating to health care. Belief in vitamin efficacy was investigated as a follow-up to the previously-cited study. We are also looking at attribution of blame by mothers for their children's medical condition with the focus on whether the blame is externalized or internalized. One of our tools is a series of projective cartoons showing a character in a variety of minor difficulties, and the mother is asked to indicate the probable cause of the misfortune. Another (somewhat more novel) projective item consists of two cartoons showing a child in bed. The child was drawn so as to give no clues as to sex, and the cartoons are identical except that one clearly shows a hospital setting, and the other is at home.

There is an additional semantic differential scale used to express attitudes towards the child's own condition. Mothers are also asked to apply items in an adjective check list to their children's behavior, and then to indicate from a list of jobs those which their children could possibly hold when they grow up. Items on both these lists are balanced between traditionally-female and traditionally-male.

In addition to the variable of sex difference, data are analyzed according to the medical condition of the child: whether congenital or acquired after birth, or whether the child is essentially "well" and has been brought to the clinic for routine examination or for treatment for some minor ailment. "Congenital" conditions included myelodysplasia, cleft lip and palate, club feet, etc. "Acquired" conditions were muscular dystrophy, juvenile rheumatoid arthritis, heart disease, orthopedic and neurological injuries.

RESULTS

(i) Attribution of Blame

An interesting observation is that, overall, mothers of boys tended to attribute blame for the cartoon characters' misfortunes to an active external agent. This was not the case with mothers of girls. Might this imply that the boys are seen as less responsible for their misfortunes, and more the prey of external causes resulting from their own active participation in life events? In any case, this was an overall finding and the source could not be attributed to any specific illness category.

The one finding with reference to ethnicity suggested that Spanish-speaking mothers tended to attribute blame for the cartoon character's misfortune more to other people than did the English-speaking Mexican Americans.

(ii) *Attribution of Blame for Their Own Children's Medical Conditions*

As might be expected, in general, more blame was externalized. However, the mothers of children with congenital conditions found a significantly greater number of external agents to blame than the others did. On an ethnic basis, both Black and Spanish-speaking mothers did more internalizing than either the Anglos or the English-speaking Mexican Americans. Once again, there appear to be two relatively homogeneous groupings: the Anglos plus English-speaking Mexican Americans on the one hand contrasted with the Spanish-speaking Mexican Americans, plus Blacks on the other. In terms of the total number of "blame items" checked, the Blacks had significantly more than the Anglos. On this measure, the other two groups were intermediate. There were no sex differences in the patterns of the attribution of blame for the medical conditions of the children.

(iii) We assumed that each mother would project the sex of her own child onto the picture of the child in bed. Such was not the case when they were presented with the picture of a child in bed at home. Although there is a tendency to identify the child in bed as the same sex as her own child, there is no significant trend. (Table I)

TABLE I
Home bed (column %)

Sex of Child

		Boy	Girl
Assigned Sex	Boy	53	49
	Girl	47	51

On the other hand, there is a significant tendency for the mother to identify with the child in the hospital bed. (See Table II)

TABLE II
Hospital bed (column %)

Sex of Child

		Boy	Girl
Assigned Sex	Boy	56	44
	Girl	44	56

On the basis of ethnicity, there were no differences in sex assignment of child in the hospital bed. There were, however, striking differences in the home bed situation. For reasons that aren't entirely clear to us yet, Anglos saw significantly more girls, and Blacks significantly more boys than the other groups, each of which made no distinction.

(iv) A semantic differential scale was used as a rating of each mother's attitude towards her own child's medical condition. Whatever the condition, it is obvious from Table III that the condition (and implicity the child) tended to be more "good" than "bad", more "whole", more "acceptable". Moreover, the children, overall, were seen as relatively healthy. There are no sex differences on the above scales.

TABLE III
"Describe your child's medical condition" (All Ss combined)

In Table IV, however, we see that although there is no distinction in judgments of "normality", the medical conditions overall are seen as more common and more ordinary for the girls. This would appear to suggest lowered expectations for their health, as compared with the boys.

TABLE IV
"Describe your child's medical condition" (All Ss combined)

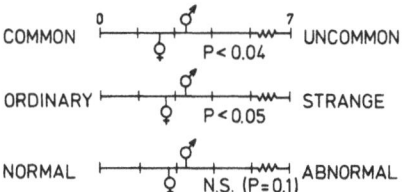

Ethnically speaking, the Spanish-speaking mothers see their children as much sicker than do the other mothers. But despite this, they are much more accepting of the child's condition than are the Blacks. Both groups see it as more normal and more common, etc. Combining six descriptive categories, we can infer that Anglos have much higher expectations for what is normal. Blacks' expectations are somewhat lower, then come English-speaking Mexican Americans, with Spanish-speaking Mexican Americans at the bottom of the scale.

(v) There were a number of ethnic differences in the attribution of sex-typed characteristics to the children. Table V summarizes the responses to the question, "Which of these words best describe your child?" Of a total of 20, an average of 7.2 were checked by each respondent. Choices were generally sex-typical (i.e., traditionally-male adjectives were applied to boys). Spanish-speaking mothers checked significantly more male adjectives than each of the other groups. This implies an importance placed on emphasizing the "macho" qualities of their boys. It should be noted that the Spanish-speaking Mexican American mothers attribute significantly fewer qualities of any kind to their girls than to their boys — an observation that is not true of any other ethnic group.

TABLE V
"Which of these words best describe your child?" (Ethnic categories)

Ethnicity	Adjective type		
	Male	Female	Total
Anglo	3.7 ⎫	3.1	6.8 ⎫
E.M.A.	3.5 ⎬ .01 ⎫	3.3	6.8 ⎬ .04
S.M.A.[a]	5.2 ⎭ ⎬ .01	2.8 ⎫ (.07)	8.0 ⎭
Black	3.7 ⎭ .01	3.6 ⎭	7.3

[a] Male-female difference was significant only for S.M.A.

(iv) In examining the issue of mothers' expectations, we looked at the question as to the jobs they considered to be potentially open to their children. Table VI shows the results according to whether the job is traditionally male of traditionally female, for all subjects combined. The overall differences resulting from matching the job expectations to the sex of the child is as to be expected. It is interesting to note, however, that there is less discrepancy based on traditionally male jobs. The suggests that girls are seen having the potential to take over "male" jobs but boys are not liable to take over jobs that are traditionally female. The difference in total job expectations based on ethnicity is presented in Table VII.

TABLE VI
"Check all the jobs your child could possibly have when he/she grows up."
(All Ss combined)

Job category	Sex of Child	
	Boy	Girl
Male job	3.9	2.0
	.01	
Female job	1.6	5.1
	.01	
Total jobs	5.5	7.1
	(.08)	

TABLE VII
"Check all the jobs your child could possibly have when he/she grows up."
(Ethnic categories)

Ethnicity	Job Category		
	Male jobs	Female jobs	Total jobs
Anglo	4.4 } .01	5.3 } .02	9.7 } .01
E.M.A.	2.3 } .01 } .01	3.3 } .01 } .01	5.6 } .01 } .01
S.M.A.[a]	1.2 } .01	0.8 } .01	1.9 } .01 } .04 } .01
Black	4.0	3.9	7.9

[a] Male-female difference was significant only for S.M.A.

IMPLICATIONS FOR HEALTH CARE

Cultural patterns vary all over the world, and although a knowledge of all inter-related aspects of a particular culture would be beneficial to the health practitioner, sex-stereotyping is of particular significance for several reasons.

First, for health practitioners, no assessment is complete without an awareness of the patient's value system. As a part of history-taking we would be well-advised to consider the relevance of sex-stereotyping and ask related questions when dealing with such pediatric problems as failure to thrive, child abuse and neglect, learning disabilities, and so forth. In the case of young children, it is their parents' values that dominate the parent/child relationship. It is necessary then to be aware of parents' health-related beliefs. Will they allow a female child to stay in bed while the male would be pushed back into the mainstream? Are males allowed to play or say they are depressed or given only aggressive vehicles such as sports for riding out critical stages in their development?

A second reason for considering sex-stereotyping is that a parent is not, as is sometimes supposed, a passive, uninformed, completely receptive part of the practitioner-patient relationship, but an active participant with his own notions about diagnosis, prognosis, and treatment. As Saunders has made clear, the parent also has ideas of how far he will go in accepting the advice and directions given by the practitioner (Saunders, 1953: 43).

A third reason that might be mentioned is that, in most Western countries, health practitioners (and especially those dealing with mental health) have also assumed the role of teacher and counselor in matters relating to children's personality and their psychoemotional growth and development.

For this reason, it is crucial to one's practice to have such culture-bound information. Where this is lacking and a parent and health practitioner do not share the same value systems or do not have an understanding that differences exist, conflicting communication and increased social distancing can occur. In other words, a prerequisite for effective communication is that those who converse must be aware of each other's assumptions and intentions (Stacey and Dearden, 1970: 26). The time in which the practitioner has to make a clinical judgment in most pediatric setting is all too brief. To make a complete and accurate assessment is difficult enough under the best of circumstances, but appropriate diagnosis and treatment are even less likely when a misunderstanding or ignorance of cultural and ethnic differences interfere with the process of communication.

CONCLUSION

Examining one's own culture-dependent behavior has the effect of sensitizing one to the behavior of others. We suggest that sex-stereotyping is one issue to be considered within a cultural context.

Health care professionals should be concerned about today's stereotyping, as it may become tomorrow's turmoil. Although we live in a pluralistic society, the practice of health care continues to be monopolistic in its relative inability to tolerate alternative systems and beliefs. If any change is to occur, one must first be willing to agree not only to the existence of, but to the value of life-patterns and belief-systems other than our own.

An understanding of ethnic differences will help us greatly in offering supportive counseling to those parents who, for lack of available folk-wisdom in their own transitional communities, seek it from us as health practitioners.

University of Southern California (M. S.)
Rancho Los Amigos Hospital (M. J.)

REFERENCES

Anderson, O.
   1963 The Utilization of Health Services. In H. Freeman et al. (eds.), Handbook of Medical Sociology. Englewood Cliffs: Prentice Hall, 349–367.
Barry, H. H., M. K. Bacon, and I. L. Child
   1957 A Cross Cultural Survey of Some Sex Differences in Socialization. Journal of Abnormal and Social Psychology 55: 327–332.
Douvan, Elizabeth
   1977 (Untitled study) cited by ISE Newsletter, Vol. 5, No. 3.
Fabrega, Horacio, Jr., and Daniel B. Silver
   1973 Illness and Shamanistic Curing in Zinacantan. California: Stanford University Press.
Fidell, Linda
   1974 Mood-modifying Drug Use in Middle Class Women. Paper presented to Western Psychological Association, Sacramento, California.
Jelliffe, D. B.
   1956 Cultural Variation and the Practical Pediatrician. The Journal of Pediatrics 45, No. 6, December.
Johnston, Maxene and Merrill Sarty
   1975 Magical Expectation in Vitamin Use. Paper presented to Western Psychological Association, Sacramento, California.
LeVine, Robert and Donald T. Campbell
   1972 Ethnocentrism: Theories of Conflict, Ethnic Attitudes, and Group Behavior. New York: John Wiley and Sons, Inc.
Mead, Margaret
   1956 Understanding Cultural Patterns. Nursing Outlook 4, No. 5, May: 260–262.
Mechanic, David
   1964 The Influence of Mothers on their Children's Health Attitudes and Behavior. Pediatrics 33: 444–453.
Mellinger, G. D., et al.
   1963 A Comparison of the Personal and Social Characteristics of High and Low Accident Children. Paper delivered at the Biennial Meeting of the Society for Research in Child Development, Berkeley, California.
Mitchell, William E.
   1977 Changing Others: The Anthropological Study of Therapeutic Systems. M. A. N. Vol. 8, No. 3, May.

Myer, R. J., et al.
  1963 Accidental Injury to the Preschool Child. Journal of Pediatrics 63: 95–105.
Rudolph, A. M.
  1977 Pediatrics. New York: Appleton-Century-Crofts.
Saunders, Lyle and Gordon Hewes
  1953 Folk Medicine and Medical Practice. Journal of Medical Education 28: 43–46.
Seward, G.
  1977 Sex Roles in Cross-Cultural Perspective. In Leonore Loeh Adler (ed.), Issues in Cross-Cultural Research. Annals of the New York Academy of Science, 612–617.
Stacey, M. and R. Dearden (eds.)
  1970 Hospitals, Children and Their Families. London: Routledge and Kegan Paul.
Torrey, E. Fuller
  1972 The Mind Game: Witchdoctors and Psychiatrists. New York: Emerson Hall Publishers.
Whiting, John W. M. and Beatrice Blyth Whiting
  1975 Altruistic and Egoistic Behavior in Six Cultures. In Laura Nader and Thomas W. Maretzki (eds.), Cultural Illness and Health. Washington: American Anthropological Association, pp. 1956–1966.
Williams, John and Susan Bennett
  1975 The Definition of Sex Stereotypes via the Adjective Check List. Sex Roles 1, No. 4: 327–337.

CAROL A. DWYER, Ph.D.

THE ROLE OF SCHOOLS IN DEVELOPING SEX ROLE ATTITUDES

I would like to discuss in this paper the role of schools and the educational process in transmitting and developing healthy attitudes toward sex roles. I will take the approach that in order for this to be accomplished, we must examine the behaviors and attitudes both of those who are educating and those who are being educated. My observations and data will be drawn from the environment with which I am most familiar, the American public education system, but I will also attempt to extend my remarks to include salient aspects of the educational systems of other cultures as I know them or have reports of them.

How Influential is Schooling?

Schools in America represent an increasingly powerful segment of the socialization process. They are the primary social agency for the transmission of cultural values as well as factual knowledge and practical skills. The schools' power stems from many sources. At the simplest, but certainly not least important, level, nearly every individual now attends school for the greatest part of the day for a period spanning twelve yars or more. In the United States today, more and more students are attending public nursery schools and pre-schools. More students than ever are now persisting in the schools through secondary school graduation, and increasing numbers are continuing on to publicly supported community colleges. Thus the time available to schools for the transmission of knowledge and values is increasing and common sense, as well as recent large-scale research projects, tells us that increased instructional time results in increased learning.

What Do Schools Teach?

Schools are now being forced to re-examine the limits of their legal and ethical responsibilities. To a large extent, parents have effectively delegated to the schools responsibility for their childrens' physical well-being; for the transmission of information and skills in the traditional academic disciplines; and for explicit instruction in vocational, social, and personal activities. Schools regularly offer guidance and training in such sex-role related areas as sex-differentiated occupations (home economics, metalworking); human sexuality and "family living"; and interpersonal relations (how to behave appropriately).

In addition to this explicit instructional activity, schools transmit implicit information on the subject of appropriate sex role behavior and attitudes. This is accomplished through a wide variety of mechanisms including sex role modeling of personal and professional characteristics (primarily on teachers); implicit

I. Gross, J. Downing, and A. d'Heurle (eds.), Sex Role Attitudes and Cultural Change, 39–43.
Copyright © 1982 by D. Reidel Publishing Company.

sex-related curricular structures (e.g., who may take what courses); implicit sex-related organizational structures (e.g., how the sexes are segregated or not); and indirect attitudinal instruction from teachers.

Public schools in the United States are forbidden by law to engage in some sex role related activities, and some structures that are interpreted as sex-discriminatory, such as separate classes for boys and girls or separate athletic teams, are now being interpreted as illegal. School personnel are now being urged to behave cautiously with regard to any actions that might be interpreted as sex-discriminatory, but the urgings and the responses are, to an overwhelming extent, simply reactive to governmental pressures. Conspicuously lacking is evidence of strong commitment, on the part of teachers or administrators, to either social or attitudinal change. Thus American public schools are becoming aware of sex-related issues, but activities stemming from this awareness are quite superficial. The major issues of sex role modeling, and sex-related patterns of achievement and motivation remain largely unexplored.

Achievement, Attitudes, and Sex Role Assumptions

In the schools' transmission of knowledge and values, the distinction between the two is often blurred. This is especially true in situations where the content of the material to be taught or learned has socially controversial or personally anxiety-producing components. Teaching about sex roles in particular is a complex net of assumptions about human behavior that are shaped by expectations that re-mold research findings, and simplify them to reduce the dissonance they create.

Educational and psychological research have made substantial contributions to our knowledge of sex-related aspect of human behavior (e.g., Maccoby and Jacklin, 1974). The research results that pertain to achievement are particularly relevant to our understanding of the schools' role in developing sex role attitudes. If we start from the premise that achievement and attitudes are interdependent (that is, that attitudes influence achievement and that achievement influences attitudes), it is necessary first to review the state of "common knowledge" about sex-related differences in achievement.

In the United States, it is an educational commonplace that girls do better in verbal areas such as reading, and boys excel in mathematics and science. Teachers and subject matter specialists, acting on these "research findings," are disinclined to question scientific verities and do not typically expend a great deal of effort to motivate girls' interest in mathematics or science, or boys' in writing or literature. In defense of teachers, this disinclination seems to be based on a feeling that trying to develop these "cross-sex" interests is in some way unnatural and therefore fruitless, rather than on any disregard for students' well-being or academic interests.

Research on sex-related patterns of achievement does not, in fact, yield any simple dichotomies of verbal and mathematical behaviors (Dwyer, 1979). One might safely say, for example, that girls of some ages and nationalities may do better on verbal tests of certain kinds than do boys of similar age and nationality. But clearly such statements are not of immense help to the educator who wishes to advise and instruct his or her students appropriately. The most appropriate generalization that can be made today about patterns of achievement is that they are highly individualized and are the product of may variables. The most clear relationship between sex and achievement is moderated by an attitudinal variable, sex role standards (Stein and Smithells, 1969; Dwyer, 1974). Sex role standards are an individual's assessment of the sex-appropriateness of various objects, activities, or behaviors. For example, a girl's sex role standard about reading would represent her personal evaluation of whether or not reading is a feminine activity. The concept of sex role standards is an important one for understanding sex-related attitudes toward achievement, for sex role standards are directly related to achievement: students perform better in those subjects that they consider sex-appropriate than in those they consider sex-inappropriate. This phenomenon seems easily explainable by dissonance theory, but more interesting work (e.g., Lockheed, 1974) suggests that some sex role standards are easily modifiable in the classroom.

We can thus expect sex role attitudes to influence achievement. These attitudes can be modified, for better or for worse, by teachers who in ordinary circumstances are passing on standards that were taught to them at home or in school. And as attitudes toward sex roles are perpetuated or modified in classroom settings we may expect to see concommitant shifts in patterns of achievement.

Other mechanisms contribute to both sex-related attitudes and achievement. The status of teachers as scholars within an educational system provides a model for students' evaluation of the sex-appropriateness of learning. The ascription of high status to teaching seems to be related to perceiving teaching as an activity suitable for males, and to enhanced learning for boys in such systems.

Schools may also alter sex role attitudes by their influence on the larger world of work. Schools have a strong influence on sex-related patterns of employment, in their capacity as certifiers of competence. Schools' guidance practices (who is steered toward what trade or profession), grading practices (how marks are awarded in various subject matter areas), and certification practices (how does one obtain the necessary credentials for a profession or for admittance to further study), are all in part reflections of the sex role standards of the educational policy makers. These standards in turn translate into facts (e.g., how many women are truly competent in mathematics?), which then further shape the attitudes of successive generations of teachers and learners.

Developing Healthy Attitudes

Healthy attitudes about sex roles cannot be meaningfully differentiated from healthy attitudes about any other subject of great importance to humanity. In most cultures, however, developing and maintaining healthy attitudes about sex roles is particularly difficult because sex roles are so closely entwined with fundamental societal structures and values, and with sexuality. For most individuals, both men and women, sex role attitudes are a fundamental part of their personalities and find expression in their daily work. If we define healthy attitudes as those characterized by flexibility and freedom of choice, we see the possibilities for schools' enhancing such attitudes. Three types of educational reform are currently taking place in the United States that I think will have the effect of producing healthier sex role attitudes. The first is legislative action forbidding sex discrimination in education. Although this legislation covers many areas of everyday life, some with conspicuously little success, the main impact appears to be in simply raising the seriousness of the issue of what is appropriate for each sex.

This legislative action is related to the second type of reform, consciousness-raising at educational policy-making and administrative levels. High-ranking educational personnel are now becoming concerned with sex equality, and the equalization of the sexes has strong implications for attitude change. The third type of reform is curricular, the development of nonsexist learning materials which stress openness and flexibility toward sex role related behavior.

These reforms are encountering serious obstacles, however. Currently among these is an under-emphasis on the impact of sex role stereotyping on men and boys. The immediate needs of girls and women have absorbed nearly all the attention of sex role attitude changers, and diverted energy from considering the burdens that unhealthy attitudes toward masculinity place on males. This is clearly related to another obstacle, the inability to differentiate sexuality and sexual behavior (physical) from sex roles (attitudinal). This common confounding puts moral and emotional blocks in the way of developing healthy sex role attitudes by diverting attention to essentially unrelated issues.

The third obstacle that I see to developing healthy sex role attitudes is over-reaction to reform. Developing healthy, sex role attitudes does not mean that women must reject those things traditionally associated with their sex, or that men must reject traditionally masculine behavior. Exchanging sex roles is a novelty with little long-term value for personal satisfaction. In a world of healthy sex role attitudes, some women will be wives and mothers, but because they have chosen to do so, not because it is inevitable. And some boys may choose to grow up and follow in the footsteps of their fathers, or may choose not to. And that freedom of choice is the essence of healthy attitudes.

Educational Testing Service, Princeton

REFERENCES

Dwyer, C. A.
  1974 The influence of children's sex role standards on reading and arithmetic achievement. Journal of Educational Psychology 66: 811–816.

Dwyer, C. A.
    1979 The role of tests and their construction in producing apparent sex-related differ-
          ences. In M. Wittig and A. Petersen (eds.), Sex-Related Differences in Cognitive
          Functioning. New York: Academic Press.
Lockheed, M.
    1974 Sex Bias in Educational Testing: A Sociologist's Perspective, (RM-74-13). Prince-
          ton, N.J.: Educational Testing Service.
Maccoby, E. E. and Jacklin, C. N.
    1974 The Psychology of Sex Differences. Stanford, Calif.: Stanford University Press.
Stein, A., and Smithells, J.
    1969 Age and sex differences in children's sex role standards about achievement.
          Developmental Psychology: 252–259.

SELMA HUGHES, Ph.D.

REVIEW OF THE LITERATURE ON NON-SEXIST CURRICULUM AND A CRITIQUE OF THE UNDERLYING ASSUMPTIONS AND RATIONALE

SUMMARY. This paper reviews the school's role in sex role socialization of young children and addresses theoretical and practical issues related to the use of non-sexist curriculum material.

INTRODUCTION

Although it has been shown by Kohlberg (1966) that children come to school already sex-typed, the influence of the school on sex role socialization is considerable. In order to place the school's impact in some perspective it is necessary to consider the course of development of sexual identity.

De Cecco et al. (1977) consider that sexual identity has four components (1) biological sex (2) gender identity (3) social sex role and (4) sexual orientation. Biological sex is the sex assigned to the child at birth. It is not always easy to determine as there may be inconsistencies between the chromosomal, hormonal, anatomical and physiological structures on which it is based. Money's work attests to the complexity yet Money (1977) points out that an individual is unable to develop a personal identity without being differentiated as masculine or feminine.

Gender identity refers to the child's basic conviction of being male or female. Kagan (1969) considers that children know their gender label by three years of age. Theorists do not agree on the way in which they acquire this conviction. Kohlberg (1966) asserts that gender identity and sexuality are not taught but result from the active structuring of experience and comprehension of physical reality. Social learning theorists postulate that it is learned through reinforcement, imitation and modeling. Maturational theorists consider psychosexual development to be a function of physiological growth and chronological age, while Hutt (1972) postulates that a biological force provides the drive for gender identity.

The third component of sexual identity is social sex role, which refers to cultural generalizations about masculinity and femininity and the normative expectations of the culture about the roles and behavior of men and women in that culture. According to Kohlberg, most children know the behavior patterns expected of them by the preschool years. Masculinity and femininity were considered independent characteristics, but behavioral scientists are now questioning the bipolar model, according to Spence and Helmreich (1978). De Cecco et al. conceptualize two independent continua of masculinity and femininity, so that an individual may possess both masculine and feminine characteristics. This concept of psychological androgyny offers a viable alternative to the

45

I. Gross, J. Downing, and A. d'Heurle (eds.), Sex Role Attitudes and Cultural Change, 45–50.
Copyright © 1982 by D. Reidel Publishing Company.

previous dichotomous choice and provides the theoretical rationale for non-sexist education.

Sexual orientation is the fourth component of sexual identity and refers to the individual's physical and affectional preference for sexual partners. Homosexuality and heterosexuality are not considered mutually exclusive by some writers, including Wolf (1978), while sexual expression is not limited to physical expression only, according to De Cecco. Psychosexual conflicts arise as children develop sexual identities and the school influences the way in which children resolve these conflicts.

ROLE OF THE SCHOOL

Lee and Gropper (1974) question whether the school serves the needs of the sexes while society undergoes changing ideas regarding sex roles. The school has the difficult task of resolving inconsistencies between the different channels of socialization, the home, the mass media, the language and the community. It is not agreed whether the school's role is to inculcate the values, customs and norms which presently prevail or to provide knowledge which could result in a transformation of those norms. There is no consensus whether teachers should "meet" children's needs in resolving problems of sexual identity or "shape" those needs, according to Guttentag and Bray (1976)

Katz (1977) succinctly summarizes recent research on sex role socialization and considers the school's role to be of three kinds (1) sex-typing effects of differences in teacher behavior toward boys and girls (2) sex-typed classroom materials and (3) the sex-typed example of its own organizational hierarchy and administrative procedures. Weitz (1977) points out that teachers also exert an indirect influence on sex role behavior which is more subtle, persuasive and difficult to combat.

There is some agreement that the schools should reexamine the restrictions and limitations imposed on boys and girls through sex bias. Many programs and policies have been challenged in the courts to break some of the sex-segregated activities. Many organizations provide data on compliance with Title IX of the Educational Amendments of 1972 which prohibits sex discrimination in education. Dunkle (1977) outlines strategies for attaining equal opportunity in competitive athletics. Sadker (1977) gives practical information on the rights of students. According to Walum (1977) sex bias against girls is more easily dissipated than that against boys. The school and the parents resist boys being associated with feminine activities.

Sex-role stereotyping in the school's instructional program has been the focus of concern for some time and is amply documented. Some of the criticisms are: boy centered stories outnumber girl centered stories; girls are depicted as passive, dependent and timid while boys are shown as active, independent and brave; males are shown in prestigious occupations while females are shown in the helping professions; math, science, social studies, spelling and reading books have been cited as sex-stereotyped, according to *Women in Words and Images* (1975), O'Donnell (1977), and Weizman and Rizzo (1974).

Many organizations have drawn up guidelines for change. The School Division of the Association of American Publishers issued a Statement on Bias-free Material (1976) and most major publishers of school texts have issued guidelines for creating positive sexual and racial images in educational materials. The National Council of Teachers of English produced guidelines to encourage the use of non-sexist language while professional organizations such as the American Psychological Association have followed suit with guidelines for non-sexist language in their journals.

It is difficult to put the proliferation of data in perspective. The public's attention continues to be drawn to sexrole stereotyping by the very vocal feminist movement. Sex bias and sex role steretyping of boys is not receiving as much attention. Frasher and Walker (1972) studied old and new editions of texts and found no change in sex roles portrayed. Graebner (1972) found an increase in the number of occupations shown for women, but male oriented stories still dominate. Guttentag and Bray (1976) found 'Sesame Street' full of sexrole stereotypes, while Gilder (1973) criticized the program for lack of sexual differentiation.

Non-sexist education is an attempt to close the gap between traditional sex roles and today's changing sex roles. Its purpose is not to obscure differences between males and females but to enable children to explore the full range of human potential. It is not the same as "unisex" and Lee (1976) states that people should be free to be and do whatever their bodies, aptitudes and interests allow. The rationale derives from the concept of psychological androgyny which Spence and Helmreich (1978) point out, is not connected to its original meaning of hermaphroditism. Bem (1974) considers that in a society where rigid sex role differentiation has outlived its utility, androgyny will come to define a more human standard of psychological health. An androgynous person may adapt more easily to different situational demands by producing the most reasonable behaviors which are required, rather than sex-related behaviors. Spence and Helmreich (1978) found that androgynous individuals display more self-esteem, social competence, and achievement orientation than individuals who are strong in either masculinity or femininity.

Several professional organizations have made a comitment to non-sexist education, e.g., the National Education Association and the Association for Childhood Education International. Many organizations have developed materials, e.g., the Resource Center on Sex Roles in Education of the National Foundation for the Improvement of Education. Many groups publish bibliographies of non-sexist books for children. Simmons (1976) warns that not every book on lists labelled non-sexist is necessarily quality literature and teachers should be alert to the dangers of self-defeating censorship. Curricula range from the trivial, to the intellectually stimulating. Activities are designed in many of the programs to draw attention to male and female sexual stereotypes, and to raise to conscious awareness, covert bias. Children are taught how to develop skills in recognizing and expressing feelings, and identifying sensitivities which both boys and girls possess. In career and vocational education, materials help children understand that one's sex need not determine one's choice of career.

There is criticism that it is difficult to translate such broad goals into specific classroom practices. Katz (1977) points out that teachers may agree in theory, but non-sexist education is difficult to implement in practice. Smelser (1977) considers that educators know what is wrong but they do not know what is right:

condemned if they attempt to produce conventional little boys and girls and condemned if they attempt some experiment in non-sexist development for the old values are far from dead. p. 279

Gilder (1973) considers the school experience damaging to the masculinity of boys and non-sexist education as a "headstart" in emasculation.

It is difficult to evaluate the impact and effectiveness of non-sexist intervention programs, for lack of criteria. Guttenag and Bray (1976) list positive outcomes of the program which they describe. Harrison (1973) concludes that the school changed through raised "consciousness", in a program in which she participated. Most programs describe increased sensitivity to sex bias and sex role stereotyping and a willingness to discuss ways of providing better educational experiences for boys and girls, as outcomes. These may not be directly related to instructional goals, but they are certainly relevant to the development of healthy attitudes towards sexuality.

CONCLUSIONS

(1) The rationale of non-sexist education appears to be sound although Walum (1977) points out that psychological androgyny needs to be investigated further to identify the conditions under which it is nourished and the conditions under which it is preferable to sex-typing.

(2) There may be age groups for which clear cut distinctions between male and female are desirable.

(3) Parents, teachers and school administrators should be aware of the issues which confront children in their search for sexual identity during a period of redefinition and realignment of social sex role. Non-sexist curricula provide a focus for awareness.

East Texas State University

REFERENCES

Association of American publishers
    1976 Statement on Bias Free Materials. AAP Office, One Park Avenue, New York, New York 10016.

Bem, S. L.
  1974 The Measurement of Psychological Androgyny Journal of Consulting and Clinical Psychology 42: 155–162.

De Cecco, J. P. and Shively, M. G.
  1977 Children's Development: Social Sex role and the Hetero-Homosexual Orientation. In Oremland, E. K. and Oremland, J. D. The Sexual and Gender Development of Young Children: The Role of the Educator. Cambridge, Mass: Ballinger Publishing Co.

Dunkle, M.
  1977 Competitive Athletics: In Search of Equal Opportunity. Washington, D. C.: National Foundation for the Improvement of Education.

Frasher, R. and Walker, A.
  1972 Sex Roles in Early Reading Textbooks. Reading Teacher 25: 741–749.

Gilder, G. S.
  1973 Sexual Suicide. New York: Bantam Books

Graebner, D. L.
  1972 A Decade of Sexism in Readers. Reading Teacher 26: 52–58.

Guttentag, M. and Bray, H.
  1976 Undoing Sex Stereotypes. New York: McGraw Hill.

Harrison, B. G.
  1974 Unlearning the Lie: Sexism in School. New York: William Morrow.

Hutt, C.
  1972 Males and Females. Harmondsworth, England: Penguin Books.

Kagan, J.
  1969 On the meaning of behavior: illustrations from the infant. Child Development 40: 1121–1134.

Katz, L. et al.
  1977 Sex Role Socialization in Early Childhood. Eric Document No. 148 472.

Katz et al.
  1977 Annotated Bibliography. Eric Document No. 148–473.

Katz, L.
  1977 Guidelines for Teachers. In Oremland, E. K. and Oremland J. D. The Sexual and Gender Development of Young Children: The Role of the Educator. Cambridge, Mass.: Ballinger Publishing Co.

Kohlberg, L.
  1966 A Cognitive developmental analysis of children's sex role concepts and attitudes. In Macoby, E. (ed.), The Development of Sex Differences. Standard, California: Standford University Press.

Lee, P. and Gropper, N.
  1974 Sex role Culture and Educational Practice. Harvard Educational Review 44: 369–410.

Lee, P.
  1976 Re-inventing Sex Roles in the Early Childhood Setting. In Growing Free. Association for Childhood Education International, 3615 Wisconsin Avenue, N. W. Washington, D. C. 20016.

Money, J.
  1977 The "Givens" from a different point of view: Lessons from Intersexuality for a theory of gender identity. In Oremland, E. K. and Oremland J. D. The Sexual and Gender Development of Young Children: The Role of the Educator. Cambridge, Mass.: Ballinger.

O'Donnell, R. W.
  1973 Sex Bias in Primary Social Studies Textbooks. Educational Leadership. 31: 137–141.

Sadker, M.
    1977 A Student Guide to Title IX. Washington, D. C.: National Foundation for the Improvement of Education.

Simmons, B.
    1976 Teachers Be(a)ware of Sex-stereotyping. In Growing Free, Association for Childhood Education International, 3615 Wisconsin Avenue, N. W. Washington, D. C. 20016.

Smelser, N.
    1977 Society's values and the educators dilemma. In Oremland, E. K. and Oremland, J. D., The Sexual and Gender Development of Young Children: The Role of the Educator. Cambridge, Mass.: Ballinger.

Spence, J. and Helmreich, R.
    1978 Masculinity and Femininity Austin, Texas: University of Texas Press.

Walum, L. R.
    1977 The Dynamics of Sex and Gender: A Sociological Perspective. Chicago: Rand McNally.

Weitz, S.
    1977 Sex Roles. New York: Oxford University Press.

Weizman, L. and Rizzo, D.
    1974 Biased Textbooks: The Images of Males and Females in Elementary School Textbooks in Five Subject Areas. Washington, D. C.: Resource Center on Sex Roles in Education.

Wolf, C.
    1978 Sex and Divided Lives. The Observer Newspaper, U.K. Sunday, 10 December.

Women on Words and Images
    1975 Dick and Jane as Victims: Sex Stereotyping in Children's Readers. Princeton, N. J.: Women on Words and Images.

SHIRLEY B. ERNST, Ph.D.

LANGUAGE AND ATTITUDES TOWARD MASCULINE AND FEMININE SEX ROLES

SUMMARY. The relationship between language and sex role concept is discussed. A review of research in which results indicate that gender generic language is, in reality, not perceived as such is presented. It is concluded that there can be no development of healthy attitudes toward masculine or feminine sex roles while language maintains the traditional stereotyped view of these roles.

INTRODUCTION

The topic of the workshop, 'How Can We Develop Healthy Attitudes Toward Masculine and Feminine Roles?' is an intriguing one since it can be treated in a variety of ways. One could discuss the concept of what is meant by "masculine" or "feminine," either from a stereotyped position or from one of the more recently emerged androgynous positions. One could look at what is meant by "healthy attitudes." The entire topic could be approached from several points of view — mental health, developmental, educational, etc. The position to be taken in this paper is that the traditional stereotypes of masculine and feminine do not lead to healthy attitudes either toward one's own sex role or toward one's own self-concept. Furthermore, certain aspects of culture, specifically the English language, support and maintain the traditional stereotyped image of masculine and feminine roles. While the basic discussion of this paper will be focused on the latter point, it is important to discuss briefly the contention that there is indeed a stereotyped view of masculine and feminine roles in contemporary society, and that these stereotypes are not healthy for members of either sex.

Much research in recent years has been centered around the topic of sex roles and the effects that stereotypes of sex roles have had on people. The results of many of these studies indicate that there are indeed common stereotypes of what is masculine and what is feminine, and that there are differing values attached to each. Iglitzin (1977) describes two studies in which she found that sex role stereotypes were held by fifth grade girls and boys. In several studies (MacBrayer, 1960; McKee and Sherriffs, 1957) results indicated that stereotyped masculine characteristics are most often seen as favorable, while stereotyped feminine characteristics are seen as unfavorable. To further compound the problem, when either males or females deviate from the stereotypical expectation for their sex, they are viewed negatively (Spence and Helmreich, 1972), thus presenting somewhat of a dilemma, particularly for members of the least favored sex (females) who aspired to be more like those of the most favored sex, (males).

Given, then, that stereotypes of what is masculine and what is feminine do exist, and that one sex is attributed more worth than the other, one should not

I. Gross, J. Downing, and A. d'Heurle (eds.), Sex Role Attitudes and Cultural Change, 51–56.
Copyright © 1982 by D. Reidel Publishing Company.

be surprised to find a variety of unhealthy attitudes in existence. Members of
the least favored sex do not value themselves, and neither are they valued by
members of the most favored sex. On the other hand, those of the most favored
sex jealously guard those attributes and behaviors which are their own, and
which are coveted by those of the less favored sex. It would seem that the more
polarized the stereotypes become, the more favor and disfavor will be attached
to the roles, thus increasing the jealously of the favored and the covetousness
of the unfavored. Therefore one could suggest that any aspect of society that
supported and maintained the stereotypes of masculine and feminine roles
would be contributing to the unhealthy attitudes developed in response to the
stereotypes.

One cultural device that seems to be responsible in part for the sex role
polarization is language, specifically the English language. The next sections of
this paper will deal with language as it is used to maintain sex role stereotypes,
and thus also to develop unhealthy attitudes towards sex roles.

GENERAL INFLUENCE OF LANGUAGE

Language has played a major role throughout human history. One aspect of the
role of language has been to preserve and transmit the traditions, values, and
attitudes of the cultural group (Capell, 1966; Chase, 1954; Luckman, 1975). As
a result of this aspect of its role, language is sometimes manipulated by a few to
benefit themselves and often harm others. May (1967) defined language used in
this way as propaganda, "an attempt to persuade people by one-sided arguments." Similarly, Allport (1954) observed that language could be misused to
develop false issues in order to form a negative attitude toward a particular
group.

History abounds with direct evidence of the influence of language on humanity. Wars have been instigated and fought, minority groups have been belittled,
and attempts have been made to wipe out whole nationalities of people with
language as the driving force and facilitators of each movement. Bosmajian
(1974) discussed several examples of successful manipulation of language. One
of these was the Vietnam war effort, where language was used to make something acceptable that ordinarily would not be so to civilized people. Another
example was Hitler's use of language to first redefine the Jews linguistically
and then to suppress and exterminate them. A third example was, and still is,
language used to maintain racial prejudice. In the case of Native Americans,
for instance, after defining the group as savages and heathens, it was a small
step toward asserting white superiority and then toward acquisition of Indian
land.

In general, the powerfulness of language is not only an influence on the
majority group, but also on the minority group which begins to accept the words
and expressions used in the stereotyping process (Podair, 1956).

SEX DIFFERENCES IN LANGUAGE

Three aspects of sex differences in language appear in the literature:

(1) differences between females and males in their use of language;

(2) differences in the way language is used to refer to women and men;

(3) the inclusionary dimensions of language, i.e. the extent to which language tends to exclude females.

While the first two aspects are both interesting and important, they are not as directly related to the topic of masculine and feminine roles as is the third point. Therefore, only the third aspect will be discussed at this time.

Exclusionary, or masculine oriented gender generic language (terms which are used to refer at times to only males and at times to both males and females, e.g. man, he, him) is used to ignore women by subsuming them into a category which is defined in terms of males. Exclusionary language has been examined and found deficient by many writers. Jespersen (1924) for example, not only described the English language as being the most "masculine" one he knew, but also pointed out the defect of exclusionary language. In addition he referred to the great amount of confusion caused by such a defect. Others (Key, 1972; Murray, 1972; Heide, 1972) have also commented similarly on the negative aspects of masculine oriented gender generic language.

It appears to an increasing number of researchers that masculine oriented generic language is not truly generic. That is, most people will not think of women when they are confronted with terms such as *men of good will, mankind*, etc. There are many empirical studies which support this point of view.

Kidd (1971) in studying the images produced by college students when pronouns were used as the generic, found that subjects did not respond to the generic pronouns as neutral. Since a significant number of subjects produced male images, Kidd concluded that the masculine pronoun as a generic does not accomplish its intended purpose, and therefore that when persons of either sex could be the antecedent, it does not suffice as a verbal indicator.

When Schneider and Hacker (1973) investigated the use of masculine oriented generic *man* with college students, they found a significantly higher number of students referring to males (by selecting pictures of males) when they were given masculine oriented labels (Social Man, Urban Man, etc.) than when they were given true generic labels (Society, Urban Life).

The extent to which junior high students visualized males and females when presented with gender-generic terms was investigated by Harrison (1975). Results indicated that students visualized predominantly more males when presented with masculine oriented generic terms (man, mankind, he) than they did when presented with terms that were inclusionary (humans, people, they; man and women, they).

In a similar study, Harrison and Passero (1975) investigated the extent to which 3rd grade children included females in their interpretation of masculine oriented generic terms. Half the children were presented with exclusionary terms (brotherhood, mankind, man-made) while the other half were presented with the neutral version of the words (community, people, hand-made). The task was to select (from four or five illustrations) and circle the appropriate drawing to illustrate the words used in a phrase or situation. On the basis of the results, the researchers concluded that children tend not to include females when presented with masculine oriented generic terms.

Nilsen (1973) investigated several aspects of grammatical gender. On one, gender as used with humanized animals, she concluded that there was a pattern of using masculine or neuter pronouns for animals with unknown sex. On another aspect, gender as related to children's perceptions of female and male roles, Nilsen found that the older the students, the closer their responses fit the stereotypes.

Ernst (1977) investigated masculine oriented generic pronouns and nouns with four hundred eighteen students ranging from pre-school through college to determine whether masculine oriented generic terms were interpreted as referring to females to the same extent as to males. Results indicated that with both the masculine oriented generic nouns and the pronouns, the receiver of the language was more likely to interpret it as referring to males than to females. For the nouns, the difference between feminine interpretations (whether the subjects thought the noun referred to females) and masculine interpretations (whether subjects thought the noun referred to males) decreased significantly when true generic nouns were used rather than masculine oriented generic nouns.

Results of each of the foregoing studies indicate that while masculine oriented generic language may be intended to include females as well as males, in reality it is not interpreted as such. In most cases, the image associated with terms such as *he* or *man* was that of a male.

DISCUSSION

If, as was suggested earlier in this paper, a society places a greater value on members of one sex than on the other, as reflected in the values of the roles and who is allowed or encouraged to perform the roles or to aspire to them, it is highly likely that negative attitudes will develop on the part of each group toward the other, as well as by one group toward itself. In a language system such as English, many masculine and feminine roles are easily identifiable. While it has been argued by some that all masculine linked terms do not refer to males alone, but rather are generic in nature, the previously discussed research indicates otherwise. If healthy attitudes toward masculine and feminine roles are to be developed, the factor of language must be given major consideration.

Many strategies have been suggested for dealing with the dilemma of sex role stereotyping through language. One suggestion has been to teach the concept of grammatical gender to children by exploring the meanings of masculine oriented generic terms (Nilsen, 1977). Other similar suggestions are contained in a publication from the National Council of Teachers of English, *Classroom Practices in Teaching English, 1976–1977: Responses of Sexism.*

While such remediation procedures are no doubt valuable, they do not address one of the basic issues. That is, as long as one sex is subsumed by language which is used to describe the other, the value of the subsumed sex is secondary. No amount of explaining that *man* also includes woman can alter the fact that *man* also defines males. Thus being male assumes a certain amount of status by not only being defined, but also by defining others.

The position is being taken in this paper that no matter what temporary measures are used to alleviate the sexism problem as it is related to language, the final solution is to correct the language itself. Language is constantly being adapted to fit the needs of a changing society. Therefore, changing language to make it more inclusionary is well within the realm of possibility. Actually what is being advocated is not really a change in language at all, but rather a change in how existing language is used. Rather than using *fireman*, for example, it would be more inclusionary as well as more correct to use the already existing term *firefighter*. Other such paired terms are in common usage: salesman-salesperson; policeman-police officer; workman-worker; mailman-letter carrier; etc. The situation with the masculine oriented pronoun, *he, his, him,* is a little more difficult since there is no matching inclusionary one. However, several techniques can be used to alleviate the situation. One can use the plural *they*, or use the *he/she* format.

No attempt is being made to claim that exclusionary language is totally responsible for the stereotyped attitudes toward sex roles. Rather, language plays a two dimensional role. It is a reflection of societal values and attitudes, while at the same time it reinforces and perpetuates the stereotypes. Certainly it is important to intervene in the cycle in ways such as providing more opportunities for non-stereotyped role attainment, and thus for non-stereotyped role modeling. However, it is also important to impact the language aspect of the cycle, thus allowing language and reality to reinforce each other in a more positive manner. Once language is not used as a tool for sex role stereotyping, the probability that people will select roles on the basis of more appropriate attributes than gender will be greatly increased. In effect, then, by removing the negative aspect of sex role stereotyping, more positive and more healthy attitudes toward sex roles will have been encouraged.

Lewis-Clark State College, Lewiston, Idaho

REFERENCES

Allport, G. W.
   1954 The Nature of Prejudice. Cambridge, Mass.: Addison-Wesley.
Bosmajian, H.
   1974 The Language of Oppression. Washington, D.C.: Public Affairs Press.

Capell, A.
	1966	Studies in Sociolinguistics. The Hague: Mouton.
Ernst, S. B.
	1977	An Investigation of Students' Interpretations of Inclusionary and Exclusionary Gender Generic Language. Doctoral dissertation. Washington State University.
Harrison, L.
	1975	Cro-Magnon woman – in eclipse. The Science Teacher 42: 8–11.
Harrison, L. and Passero, R. N.
	1975	Sexism in the language of elementary school textbooks. Science and Children 12: 22–25.
Heide, W. S.
	1972	The sine qua non for a just society. Vital Speeches 38: 403–409.
Iglitzin, L. B.
	1977	A child's eye view of sex roles. In Sex Role Stereotyping in the Schools. National Education Association, Washington, D. C.
Jespersen, O.
	1924	The Philosophy of Grammar. London: George Allen and Unwin.
Key, M. R.
	1972	Linguistic behavior of male and female. Linguistics 88: 15–31.
Kidd, V.
	1971	A study of the images produced through the use of the male pronoun as the generic. Moments in Contemporary Rhetoric and Communication 1(2): 25–29.
Luckman, T.
	1975	The Sociology of Language. Indianapolis: Bobbs-Merrill.
MacBrayer, C. T.
	1960	Differences in perception of the opposite sex by males and females. Journal of Social Psychology 52: 309–314.
May, F. B.
	1967	Teaching Language as Communication to Children. Columbus, Ohio: Charles E. Merrill.
McKee, J. P. and Sherriffs, A. C.
	1957	The differential evaluation of males and females. Journal of Personality 25: 356–371.
Murray, J.
	1972	Male perspective in language. Women, A Journal of Liberation 3: 46–50.
National Council of Teachers of English
	1977	Classroom Practices in Teaching English, 1976–1977: Responses to Sexism. Urbana, Illinois: NCTE.
Nilsen, A. P.
	1973	Grammatical gender and its relationship to the equal treatment of males and females in children's books. Doctoral dissertation, University of Iowa.
Nilsen, A. P.
	1977	In defense of teaching the concept of grammatical gender. In Classroom Practices in Teaching English, 1976–1977: Responses of Sexism. Urbana, Illinois: NCTE.
Podair, S.
	1956	Language and prejudice toward Negroes. Phylon 17: 390–394.
Schneider, J. and Hacker, S.
	1973	Sex Role Imagery and use of the generic "man" in introductory texts: a case in the sociology of sociology. American Sociologist 8: 12–18.
Spence, J. T. and Helmreich, R.
	1972	Who likes competent women: competence, sex role congruence of interests, and subjects' attitudes toward women as determinants of interpersonal attraction. Journal of Applied Social Psychology 2: 197–213.

ALICE D. GROSS, Ed.D.

DOES SEX STEREOTYPING LEAD TO A HIGHER INCIDENCE OF MALE DYSLEXIA?

SUMMARY. Inconsistent and contradictory findings across cultures, with respect to *sex differences* in *dyslexia* raise doubts about physiological explanations for this male-prevalent condition. Additional doubts are raised due to recent disclosures of sexist bias in determining who shall be labeled as dyslexic.

The intent of this comparative study is to attempt to clarify the roles attributed to physiological differences between males and females as putative causes of dyslexia and the impact of sex-role socialization and comprehensive health services on the male prevalence of this condition.

The particular comparative cultures will be a Kibbutz population and a Moshav population in the state of Israel. A Kibbutz is a communal settlement where production, consumption and childrearing are collectivized. A Moshav is a settlement of families where only production is collectivized. These populations are most appropriate to test hypotheses about sex differences because of the wide variation their socialization structures represent; from collective childrearing with a similar socialization, to familistic childrearing with sex-differentiated socialization. Non-biased prevalence data on dyslexia will be collected.

INTRODUCTION

Of all the disabilities noted with unequal sex ratios, dyslexia exhibits the greatest disparity. The ratio averages ten boys per girl (Mumpower, 1970; Wyatt, 1966; Durrell, 1965; Bentzen, 1963). The purported phenomenon of female reading superiority is also buoyed by an overwhelming body of evidence (Stanchfield, 1971, Dykstra and Tinney, 1969; Gates, 1961). More recent disclosures of this disparity is found in Maccoby and Jacklin's *Psychology of Sex Differences* (1974). Following the two authors' painstaking reexamination and debunking of most purported sex differences, they conclude that male dominance in dyslexia has been solidly established and is a consequence of the male organism's vulnerability to pathology.

Such overwhelming evidence of higher incidence of dyslexia among males helps us understand the uncritical acceptance of the assertion that male dyslexia is determined by the physiological make-up of the male. Furthermore, one must read the convincing case made by Bentzen, 1963; Garai, 1971, Hutt, 1972 and Buffery and Gray, 1972. A review of this literature may easily lead one to conclude that a physiological basis does exist for male dyslexia. However, contradictory findings from an Israeli Kibbutz system (Gross, 1977) reported by this investigator at the last World Congress raise doubts about explanations that exclude cultural variables.

In general, Kibbutz findings did not lend support to the three prominent physiological explanations offered for male dyslexia. They are "maturational

I. Gross, J. Downing, and A. d'Heurle (eds.), Sex Role Attitudes and Cultural Change, 57–64.
Copyright © 1982 by D. Reidel Publishing Company.

lag"; "crossed dominance" and the "vulnerability of the male organism." Specifically, no gender differences were found in percentage of dyslexic cases and in the area of reading performance level. In fact, both boys and girls performed at the same high percentile rankings for Israeli norms derived for evaluation of reading performance. Crossed-dominance, maturational lag and twelve other indices of psychopathology were not found related to sex nor to cases of male dyslexia. However, one relationship supported by the data analyses was that of sex-role standards and reading performance. Both sexes considered reading as a sex-appropriate activity. Perhaps these findings indicate that even if physiological factors may exert an influence on the emergence of dyslexia it is equally possible that cultural factors may render them inoperative. It is the intent of this proposed comparative study to investigate this possibility further through the roles played by similar sex role socialization and comprehensive health services. With respect to the latter, this service is readily accessible to all Kibbutz members and may, through pre- and post-natal care, protect the more vulnerable male from expressing its greater vulnerability to dyslexia.

All the evidence cited for the existence of this sex-related component of dyslexia is derived from incidence data. These data originate primarily from one cultural source; American clinics and the American school systems. According to Hobbs (1975) American incidence data is unreliable due to a sexist bias operating to refer greater number of boys than girls. Most American researchers do not differentiate those aspects of dyslexia which may be culture specific from those which may be physiological in origin. Such an omission, they explain, is inevitable until such time as boys and girls can be socialized in the same way. "Whatever the 'real' differences between the sexes may be, we are not likely to know them until the sexes are treated differently, that is alike," (Kate Millet, *Sexual Politics*, p. 29). Fortunately within the Kibbutz Artzi system boys and girls are socialized similarly (Rabin, 1967; Bettleheim, 1969; Rabin and Hazan, 1973).

Sex Role Standards and Early Sex Role Socialization. Kibbutz studies imply that the system of collective childrearing that intentionally advocates similar sex role socialization results in perception of reading as a sex appropriate activity for boys and girls. Some American studies indicate that sex role standards might provide a means for understanding and contribute to an explanation for the differential in dyslexia. According to these studies, American boys' preception of reading, as well as other school related activities, are feminine, and therefore inappropriate to, or in conflict with, their masculine identification. Such a dissonant situation, they suggest, depresses boys reading performance. Among the studies which advocate for this position are: Mazurkiewicz, 1959; Coleman, 1961; Lamkin, 1967; Kagan, 1969; Stein and Smithells, 1969 and Tregaskis, 1972.

Maccoby (1974) suggests that any direct attempt to modify sex role standards in relation to intellectual functioning including reading, may prove futile while changes in upbringing that affect certain central personality characteristics may have the desired effect. Maccoby links sex role standards to early sex role socialization. Three-year olds have already developed differentiated toy preferences and have learned that there are activities and duties appropriate for each sex and that they prefer to play with same sex children (Kohlberg, 1966; Nadelman, 1974; Thompson, 1975).

The major summarizing papers on children's development of sex role standards are: Kagan, 1964; R. Sears et al., 1965; Kohlberg, 1966; Mussen, 1969 and Mischel, 1970. All emphasize the roles played by imitation and identification of the sex-differentiated adult world, as represented by parents, media and adults in general. Such explanations are not sufficient to explain Kibbutz children's acquisition of similar sex role standards and their ready engagement in cross-sex activities in comparison with their non-Kibbutz counterparts. The adult work world of Kibbutz is as sex-differentiated as the non-Kibbutz world (Shepher, 1975). The sex stereotypes projected by Israeli media enter the Kibbutz as readily as it enters other aspects of the Israeli culture. Perhaps a more plausible explanation might be that all children learn both masculine and feminine behaviors through observation. However, only the Kibbutz culture provides the critical conditions necessary to express cross-sex behavior, through its intentional ideological advocacy for similar sex role standards (Rabin, 1969) and its offer of such opportunities among its children. Perhaps the society's sex role ideology concomitant with practices of the childrens' primary socializing agents are significant shapers of children's reading abilities.

METHOD

This research will compare two communal settings in Israel, namely, the Moshav and the Kibbutz. These populations form an excellent match for comparative study; they share many points of commonality in organization and cooperative features. However, the Moshav still retains economic dependence on the nuclear family in which children are raised. The father is the traditional head of the family and mothers' responsibilities are for childrearing and household chores. As in the Kibbutz, comprehensive health services are available without charge to the family (Weintraub, 1969; Baldwin, 1971).

The specific questions to be studied are whether or not the results of an earlier study (Gross, 1977) reported at the 1978 World Congress reflect the non-sexist collective childrearing in the Artzi Kibbutzim or may reflect a more general aspect of the Israeli society? In an attempt to address these questions the study performed with the Kibbutz population will be expanded and replicated with a Moshav population.

Overview of Research Plan. Fifty children of each sex will be selected randomly in nursery school, second, fifth and seventh grades respectively. The four-year olds and kindergarteners will be tested on pre-reading skills and with respect to sex role standards for reading. The older children will be given tests of general reading performance, sex role standards for reading, crossed dominance, and their records will be reviewed with regard to twelve indices of psychopathology as well as for classification as superior readers and as dyslexics. In addition to teacher certification for reading problems the standardized reading tests will be used to confirm this diagnosis. The use of the Bender Gestalt for the younger children is to provide an index of maturation level.

DISCUSSION

The intent of this study is not to disprove the inferred causal nature of physiological factors in male dyslexia, but rather, to point out that in certain cultures the influence of such factors may be inoperative. If the results of this study confirm the findings of my study reported at the 1978 World Congress, the position that high reading performance for both sexes occurs within a non-sexist socialization system, then such evidence should give us pause to reconsider prevailing theories and practices. The restrictive effects of sex stareotyping on boys and girls have only recently become recognized (Bem and Bem, 1970). There is abundant evidence from Western cultures that parents encourage their children to develop restrictive sex-typed interests (Maccoby and Jacklin, 1974). Even more to the point is the fact that parents actively discourage their children, particularly their sons, from engaging in activities they consider appropriate only for the opposite sex (Hartup and Moore, 1963; Fling and Manosevitz, 1972). It appears that this reaction stems from the fear that 'feminine' behavior in a boy is likely to be construed as an indication of homosexual tendencies (Maccoby, 1974). It is interesting to note that in three generations of collective experience in Kibbutz childrearing no cases of homosexual preference has been reported (Neubauer, 1965; Zellermeyer and Marcus, 1972).

One goal of this research will have been achieved if it serves to stimulate parents and other socializing agents to become aware of the effects of sex-stereotyping on learning. It is difficult to effect changes in belief systems unless those beliefs are a matter of public debate. Before this debate can be joined, stereotyped thinking must be brought into conscious awareness. The ultimate goal of such research is to promote the development of more competent and healthier human beings.

University of Rhode Island

TABLE I
Grade and sex distribution and test instruments used in a Moshav population

Grade	Boys	Girls	Marginal Totals	Instruments to be Administered
Nursery School	50	50	100	Bender Gestalt: Sex Role Standards Test
Kindergarten	50	50	100	Bender Gestalt: Sex Role Standards Test
Second Grade a. Superior readers b. Dyslexics	50	50	100	Reading Test; Sex Role Standards Test; Crossed Dominance Test; Individual Diagnoses for 12 psycho-pathologies
Fifth Grade a. Superior readers b. Dyslexics	50	50	100	
Seventh Grade a. Superior readers b. Dyslexics	50	50	100	
	250	250	500 = Total Sample Population	

TABLE II
Grade and sex distribution and test instruments used in a Kibbutz population

Grade	Boys	Girls	Marginal Totals	Instruments to be Administered
Nursery School	50	50	100	Bender Gestalt; Sex Role Standards Test
Seventh Grade a. Superior readers b. Dyslexics	50	50	100	Reading Test; Sex Role Standards Test; Crossed Dominance Test; Individual Diagnoses for 12 psycho-pathologies
	100	100	200 = Total Sample Population	

62   ALICE D. GROSS

REFERENCES

Anthony, E. James.
1970 Behavior Disorders. In P. H. Mussen (ed.), Manual of Child Psychology. New York: John Wiley and Sons: 667–764,

Baldwin, Elaine
1975 Differentiation and Cooperation in an Israeli Veteran Moshav. Manchester: Manchester University Press.

Bem. D. and Bem, S.
1970 We're All Non-conscious Sexists. In D. J. Bem (ed.), Beliefs, Attitudes and Human Affairs. Belmont, Calif.: Brooks/Cole.

Bentzen, Frances
1963 Sex Ratios in Learning and Behavior Disorders. American Journal of Orthopsychiatry 33: 92–98.

Bettleheim, Bruno
1969 The Children of the Dream. New York: Macmillan Co., 1969.

Buffery, Anthony and Gray, J. A.
1972 Sex Differences in the Development of Spatial and Linguistic Skills. In Ounsted, Christopher and Taylor, David C. (eds.), Gender Differences: Their Ontogeny and Significance. Edinburgh and London: Livingstone: 123–157.

Coleman, James S.
1961 The Adolescent Society. New York: The Free Press of Glencoe.

Durrell, Donald
1956 Improving Reading Instruction. New York: Harcourt Brace and World.

Dwyer, Carol A.
1974 Influence of Children's Sex Role Standards on Reading and Arithmetic Achievement. Journal of Educational Psychology 66 (December): 811–816.

Fling, S. and Manosevitz, M.
1972 Sex Typing in Nursery School Children's Play Interests. Developmental Psychology 7: 146–152.

Garai, J. E.
1970 Sex Differences in Mental Health. Genetic Psychology Monographs 81: 123–142.

Gross, Alice D.
1977 The Relationship between Sex Differences and Reading Ability in an Israeli Kibbutz System. In Feitelson, Dina (ed.), Cross-Cultural Perspectives in Reading and Reading Research. Newark, Delaware: The International Reading Assoication. 72–88.

Gross, Alice D.
1978 Sex Role Standards and Reading Achievement. The Reading Teacher 32 (November): 149–156.

Hartup, W. W. and Moore, S. G.
1963 Avoidance of Inappropriate Sex Typing by Young Children. Journal of Consulting Psychology 27: 467–473.

Hobbs, Nicholas
1975 The Future of Children: Categories, Labels and Their Consequences. San Francisco, Calif.: Jossey Bass.

Hutt, Corinne
1972 Sex Differences in Human Development. Journal of Human Development 15: 153–170.

Kagan, Jerome
1964 The Child's Sex Role Classification of School Objects. Child Development 35: 1051–1056.

Kagan, Jerome
   1969 Sex Typing during the Pre-School and Early School Years. In Janis, Irving, et al.
         (eds.), Personality Dynamics, Development and Assessment. New York: Harcourt,
         Brace and World.
Kohlberg, L.
   1966 A Cognitive Developmental Analysis of Children's Sex Role Concepts and Atti-
         tudes. In Maccoby, E. (ed.), The Deyelopment of Sex Differences. California:
         Standord University Press.
Lamkin, Floyd D.
   1967 Masculinity-Femininity of Pre-Adolescent Youth in Relation to Behavior Accept-
         ability, Tested and Graded Achievement, Inventoried Interests and General
         Intelligence. Unpublished Doctoral dissertation, University of Virginia.
Maccoby, Eleanor E.
   1966 Sex Differences in Intellectual Functioning. In Maccoby, Eleanor (ed.), The
         Development of Sex Differences. Standford, Calif.: Standford University Press.
Maccoby, Eleanor, E. and Jacklin, Carol N.
   1974 The Psychology Sex Differences. Standford, Calif.: Standord University Press.
MacFarlane, Jean W., Allen, L., and Honzik, M.
   1954 A Developmental Study of the Behavior Problems of Normal Children between
         21 Months and 14 Years. Child Development 2.
Mazurkiewicz, Albert J.
   1959 Social Cultural Influences and Reading. Journal of Developmental Reading 3
         (Summer): 254–263.
Millet, Kate
   1969 Sexual Politics. New York: Avon Books.
Mischel, W.
   1970 Sex Typing and Socialization. In Mussen, P. H. (ed.), Carmichael's Manual of
         Child Psychology. New York: Wiley.
Mumpower, D. L.
   1970 Sex Ratios Found in Various Types of Referred Exceptional Children. Excep-
         tional Children 23 (April): 621–626.
Mussen, P. H.
   1969 Early Sex Role Development. In Goslin, D. A. (ed.), Handbook of Socialization
         Theory and Research. Chicago: Rand McNally.
Nadelman, L.
   1974 Sex Identity in American Children: Memory, Knowledge and Preference Tests.
         Developmental Psychology 10: 413–417.
Neubauer, Peter (ed.)
   1965 Children in Collectives: Child Rearing Aims and Practices of the Kibbutz. Spring-
         field, Ill.: Charles C. Thomas.
Rabin, Albert I.
   1965 Growing Up in a Kibbutz. New York: Springer.
Rabin, Albert I. and Hazan, Bertha
   1973 Collective Education in the Kibbutz. New York: Springer.
Sear, R. R., et al.
   1965 Identification and Child Rearing. California: Standord University Press.
Shepher, Joseph
   1969 Familism and Social Structure: The case of the Kibbutz. Journal of Marriage and
         the Family 31: 567–573.
Stein, Althea H. and Smithells, Jancis
   1969 Age and Sex Differences in Children's Sex Role Standards about Achievement.
         Developmental Psychology 1: 252–259.

Thompson, S. K.
    1975 Gender Labels and Early Sex Role Development. Child Development 16: 339–
          347.
Tregaskis, Egor K.
    1972 The Relationship between the Sex Role Standards of Reading and Reading
          Achievement of First Grade Boys. Unpublished Doctoral dissertation, State
          University of New York at Albany.
Weintraub, Dov, et al. (ed.)
    1969 Moshava, Kibbutz and Moshav: Patterns of Jewish Rural Settlement and Develop-
          ment in Palestine. Ithaca: Cornell University Press.
Wyatt, Nita M.
    1966 The Reading Achievement of First Grade Boys vs First Grade Girls. Reading
          Teacher 19 (May): 661–665.
Zellermayer, Julius and Marcus, Joseph
    1972 Kibbutz Adolescence: Relevance to Personality Development Theory. Journal of
          Youth and Adolescence 1, No. 2: 143–153.

JOHN DOWNING, Ph.D.

MAKING LITERACY EQUALLY ACCESSIBLE TO FEMALES AND MALES

INTRODUCTION

In his survey of literacy customs in traditional societies, Goody (1968) found evidence of many social influences on the extent of literacy within cultures. For example, a very common cause of restriction on literacy has been the preservation of secrecy as in religious or magical books. Goody concluded that "such restrictive practices tend to arise wherever people have an interest in maintaining a monopoly of the sources of their power" (p. 12). In this paper, I shall attempt to show how restrictive practices continue to discriminate between the sexes regarding the accessibility of literacy and I shall suggest some ways that may lead to greater equity in this respect.

SEX DIFFERENCES IN LITERACY LEVELS

Nearly all American investigations, among the more important being those of Samuels (1943), Carroll (1948), Prescott (1955), and Anderson, Hughes and Dixon (1957), show significant differences between boys and girls on reading readiness measures in favor of the girls, though one or two other investigators, for example Potter (1949), and Konski (1955), found no significant differences. American research also shows quite clearly that in that country girls have a superiority over boys in the acquisition of reading skill (Durrell, 1940; Alden, Sullivan and Durrell, 1941; Gates, 1961; and Dykstra and Tinney, 1969).

In the past, before comparisons began to be made with other countries, it was usually assumed that this difference between the sexes that had been found in the American studies was a universal human characteristic, and explanations were sought in terms of a differential rate or level of maturation in girls as compared with boys. The modern more skeptical view of the differential maturation hypothesis is summed up in this conclusion from Harris and Sipay: "It would seem possible, therefore, that sex differences are due more to school-related factors than to biological factors" (p. 20).

But the school is a cultural institution and, therefore, we should anticipate that these "school-related factors" may vary from one culture to another. Hence it is not surprising that, when one compares different countries, one finds contrasting patterns of differences between the sexes in their reading achievements. In some countries the opposite result to the American finding has been reported. Boys were found to have superior reading achievements to girls in Nigeria (Abiri, 1969), India (Oommen, 1973), Germany (Preston, 1962), and Finland (Viitaniemi, 1965). In England, which would be expected to share some

65

I. Gross, J. Downing, and A. d'Heurle (eds.), Sex Role Attitudes and Cultural Change, 65–79.
Copyright © 1982 by D. Reidel Publishing Company.

common linguistic and cultural variables with America, there have been conflicting findings on this question but this conflict of evidence is, at least, contrary to the general agreement in American research that girls are at an advantage over boys in beginning reading (Thackray, 1965, 1971; Ministry of Education, 1950, 1957; Morris, 1966; Pringle, Butler and Davie, 1966). If one may generalize at all from these conflicting results, the conclusion would appear to be that in England there is a rather weak trend for girls to achieve better in reading than boys on average, but that the difference between the sexes is quite unimportant.

The above mentioned studies, with the exception of Preston's (Germany/U.S.A.), were not comparative but one investigation does provide comparable statistics from objective testing in several different countries. Johnson (1973–1974) administered the same English language reading attainment test in Canada, England, Nigeria and the United States. Only in Canada and the United States was there a clear superiority for the female samples. In Nigeria the males were significantly ahead. In England the boys also had an overall advantage, but the results were more mixed on the various subtests.

SEX DIFFERENCES IN THE TREATMENT OF READING DISABILITY

Many studies have found that boys outnumber girls in treatment centers for reading disability. For example, in questioning Preston's German findings, Orlow (1976) has shown that many more boys than girls suffer from *Legasthenie* (dyslexia) in Germany. Research statistics confirm a similar trend elsewhere. For example, Schonell (1942) in a survey of 15,000 London school children, found that 5 per cent of boys and 2.5 per cent of girls were retarded in reading development by 1.5 years or more. The Ministry of Education (1950) survey for England found about twice as many boys as girls were in the lowest category of "illiterate".

When one examines the statistics for cases referred to clinics the difference between the sexes appears even more remarkable. Monroe (1932) and Blanchard (1936) each independently reported that 86 per cent of their reading disability cases were boys. Fernald's (1943) cases were 97 per cent boys, and Young (1938) had 90 per cent boys among 41 reading disabled cases.

The theory that specific reading disability or dyslexia is a sex-linked hereditary condition is found in almost every text on dyslexia. For example, Critchley (1970) in support of that theory writes: "Of my own 616 cases referred to me as potential dyslexics, and personally examined, 487 were males and 129 were females" (p. 91). Miles (1974) states as evidence for his theory that dyslexia is constitutionally determined "the fact that it is more common in boys than in girls" (p. 86). Similarly Crosby (1969) claims that "dyslexia . . . occurs three to four times as frequently among males as females" (p. 10).

Eisenberg (1966) gives a somewhat different biological explanation of the apparent greater susceptibility of males to reading disability. He writes that, "It would seem more appropriate to relate these disproportions to the greater biological vulnerability of the male to a wide variety of ills; from the moment of conception onwards, there is a highly significant differential in morbidity and mortality between the sexes . . . " (p. 15).

But all of these 'facts' about sex differences in reading disability relate to *referrals* not to surveys of the population of males and females. Information about children referred for treatment tell us only about the *incidence* of reading disability or dyslexia among boys and girls who were *selected* for treatment. This selection could be affected by prejudiced opinions or unconscious attitudes toward sex differences in literacy needs. For example, Vernon (1957) proposed that,

Perhaps the most likely explanation . . . is that the reading disability cases in boys often have emotional disorders in addition, and these are frequently agressive disorders. Thus the boys are referred to clinics because these disorders, rather than the disability, have brought them to the notice of teachers and parents (p. 114).

An unusual opportunity to study the prevalence of reading disability among unselected boys and girls in the general population instead of its incidence in those selected for special treatment occurs in the Israeli kibbutz system. There equality of the sexes is a fundamental principle. A conscious effort is made to treat boys and girls alike. The possibility of studying differences between boys' and girls' behavior in the kibbutz system is good because observational and test records are kept routinely on all the children from an early age. Gross (1978) studied a sample of 305 kindergartners, second graders and fifth graders randomly selected from a population of 1,871 kibbutz children at these grade levels. She found no significant differences between the sexes in reading performance. Furthermore, "No gender differences were evident in percentage of reading disability cases. Thirteen per cent of both boys and girls were found to be reading disabled (13 out of 102 boys, 12 out of 96 girls)." Even more pertinent to Eisenberg's claim was Gross' finding that, "crossed dominance, maturational lag, and 12 additional indices of psychopathology were found to be unrelated to cases of male reading disability" (p. 153). Gross' results raise doubts about theories that boys are necessarily at a disadvantage in learning to read because of their biological sex. They also raise the suspicion that *sex role prejudices are influencing the diagnosis of dyslexia and reading disability*.

SEX ROLE STEREOTYPES ABOUT READING

One mechanism that may be effective in making reading instruction less accessible to boys in America seems to be indicated by the research of Samuels and Turnure (1974). They used a behavioral observation schedule to investigate sex differences in classroom attentiveness and its relation to reading achievement among a sample of American first grade boys and girls. They found that the girls were significantly more attentive than boys during the reading period, and that "increasing degrees of attention were related to superior word recognition"

(p. 31). Samuels and Turnure relate this finding to that of Cobb and Hops (1973) that overt task-relevant orienting behavior is connected with scholastic achievement. Samuels and Turnure conclude that "the sex difference favoring girls frequently found in reading achievement seems to be mediated by an attentional variable" (p. 31).

Why should these American girls have been more attentive than the American boys in this study by Samuels and Turnure? A probable answer is suggested by what Dwyer (1973) refers to as *"cultural expectations for the male sex role*. Boys' perceptions of school and the reading activity as inappropriate to or in conflict with development of the male sex role may depress boys' achievement" (p. 455). Dwyer's concept of "cultural expectations" refers to the *source* of students' perceptions of what behavior is appropriate for their sex roles. The *actual perceptions themselves* are often referred to as "sex role standards" (Kagan, 1964). Thus the *cultural expectations* held by adults and older children influence the development of *sex role standards* in younger members of the culture.

Stein and Smithells (1969) found that reading activities are popularly regarded as feminine in the United States and Downing and Thomson (1977) concluded similarly in their investigation in Canada. A recent study by Downing and an international team of educational researchers (1979) investigated cultural expectations and sex role standards about reading in Canada, Denmark, England, Finland, Israel, Japan, and U.S.A.

THE PRESENT INVESTIGATION

Aims

The research reviewed above suggests that sex role standards derived from cultural expectations may have an important influence on reading achievements. Some of the other research reviewed above indicates that the pattern of sex differences in reading achievement varies from country to country. Therefore, it may be predicted that cultural expectations and sex role standards may differ between countries.

The hypothesis tested in this present research was that cultural expectations and sex role standards within one country would be congruent but that they would differ between countries. The countries to be compared were Canada, Denmark, England, Finland, Israel, Japan, and U.S.A.

Tests

It was thought that the problem of translating a verbal questionnaire into the different languages of these countries could be avoided by developing a picture test. Each subject was presented with an 'Object' booklet and an 'Activity' booklet. Each booklet contained two sample pictures for practice and ten operational drawings as the test items. The 'Object' booklet contained pictures of things that might be appropriate as gifts for boys or girls of about six years of age. The two critical test items were drawings of books, one in an open face position and the other closed, standing on its edge. The other items were included to mask the focus of the investigation on reading. The 'Activity' booklet contained drawings of a neuter 'stick' person engaging in various activities with the same operational items as shown in the 'Object' booklet. Each activity depicted could be characteristic of a boy or girl of about six years of age. Two of the 'Activity' pictures were of the 'stick' child reading, one lying down and the other seated in a chair. The purpose of these critical items also was masked by the other irrelevant items.

In addition, to the right of each item in both booklets, were placed two drawings intended to be obviously a boy and a girl respectively. The subject's task was to circle the boy if the object or activity was perceived as being more appropriate for boys, or to circle the girl if the item was seen as more appropriate for girls. The forced-choice method was used. The subject had only two choices either the boy or the girl.

The code letters either 'G' or 'B' were printed on the covers of the booklets according to whether they were to be given to either female or male subjects respectively. Each individual subject's pair of booklets had the same alphanumeric coding on their covers. The collaborators in the various countries investigated reviewed the booklets in a pilot study and some modifications were made to insure comparable understanding by subjects in all countries.

The Sample

The sampling plan for each country was designed to approximate as closely as possible to the demographic characteristics of the model sample selected in Canada. The aim was to obtain six sub-samples in every participating country:

1. *The adult public*: Starting from a table of random numbers a sample of approximately 200 subjects was drawn from the electoral roll of one municipality (a different municipality from the one studied in the earlier investigation by Downing and Thomson). Interviewers were given a list of names and addresses. Only these persons listed could be interviewed. If any of them had moved away, died, or refused to cooperate, the interviewer had to take the next name on the list of reserve subjects which had been selected by the random procedure described.

2. *Education students*: The complete population of second year Education students at the University of Victoria was tested.

3. *Grade I pupils* (age 6 plus): 100 pupils in four classes selected to be typical in

home background for the school district (a mixed suburban/rural area at one side of an urban centre with about 100,000 population.

4. *Grade IV pupils* (age 9 plus): 100 pupils chosen by the same method.

5. *Grade VIII pupils* (age 13 plus): 100 pupils chosen by the same method.

6. *Grade XII pupils* (age 17 plus). 100 pupils chosen by the same method.
    Similar sub-samples were sought in Denmark, England, Finland, Israel, Japan, and U.S.A.

Procedure

All interviewers participated in a training workshop in the interviewing methods to follow. They also conducted two pilot interviews and the results and any problems encountered were discussed at a second workshop session.

In the sample of the adult public subjects were interviewed in their own homes. Each interviewer carried an official letter of authorization. After a brief introduction the standard instructions were given. These explained that the research was about the kinds of things young boys and girls should have and the kinds of activities that were more suitable for girls or for boys. The subject was asked to

think of the average boy aged about six and the average girl of about six years of age as well. For example, the first picture is a toy truck and the second is a doll. We would like you to draw a circle round the little boy if you think the thing is more suitable to give to a little boy, or draw the circle round the girl if you feel that it would make a better gift for a little girl. There are no right or wrong answers to our questions. We just want to know what you think is better. Please draw only one circle on each page. If it is difficult to decide just make a quick guess, please. Would you try the first two pages, please?

Further explanations were given if necessary. Then the interviewer continued:

Now may we have your opinion about the other things in the book. Just decide if it would be better to give the thing to a little boy or a little girl. Please draw one circle only around either the little boy or the little girl on each page.

The instructions for the Activity booklet were similar. The order of presentation of the two booklets was reversed in half the cases to control for bias due to the order of response options. The explanations were abbreviated for whichever booklet was presented second.

The college and school student samples were tested as whole classes. To insure that the subjects' responses could be proctored to see that they were following the correct procedure at least two interviewers worked together in administering the group tests. One of these read out the standard instructions which were parallel to those used in the individual interviews already described. One half of the subjects received the Object booklet first. The other half received the Activity booklet first. Precautions were taken to insure that every item in the booklets had been completed in every individual or group interview.

In Denmark, Finland, Israel, and Japan, respectively, the standard interview instructions were translated into Danish, Finnish, Hebrew and Japanese.

RESULTS

Sampling

It proved impossible to obtain all six sub-samples in some of the countries. Denmark could not obtain a sample of college students. The adult public sample was not obtainable in Israel, Japan, and the U.S.A. Grade 12 students were not obtained in Israel. A further unavoidable difficulty was the variability in the age and grade levels studied in the different countries. However, in each country a developmental cross section was made that can be described in terms of six levels:

Level 1: Canada – grade I (age 6); Denmark – nursery school (age 6); England – first year infants (age 5); Finland – grade I (age 7); Israel – grade I (age 6); Japan – grade I (age 6); U.S.A. – grade I (age 6).

Level 2: Canada – grade IV (age 9); Denmark – grade III (age 9); England – second year juniors (age 9); Finland – grade IV (age 10); Israel – grade IV (age 9); Japan – grade IV (age 9); U.S.A. – grade IV (age 9).

Level 3: Canada – grade VIII (age 13); Denmark – grade VI (age 12); England – second year secondary (age 13); Finland – grade VIII (age 14); Israel – grade VIII (age 13); Japan – grade VII (age 12); U.S.A. – grade VIII (age 13).

Level 4: Canada – grade XII (age 17); Denmark – grade X (age 16); England – first year sixth form (age 17); Finland – grade XII (age 18); Israel – not represented; Japan – grade X (age 15); U.S.A. – grade XII (age 17).

Level 5: college students of education in all countries except Denmark.

Level 6: adults in Canada, Denmark, England and Finland only. In Denmark the sampling procedure described earlier proved difficult. Therefore, testing had to be performed at adult education centers.

The number of subjects in each sub-sample is given in Tables I and II. Data from levels 1 through 4 were related to children's sex role standards. Data from levels 5 and 6 were obtained to provide information on cultural expectations.

Sex Role Standards and Expectations

Figure 1 and 2 summarize the percent of female and male subjects respectively
who responded "girl" at each level. These percentages were obtained by pooling
all the responses on the four critical items of the test. These percentages are
listed in Tables I and II.

To test for the statistical significance of the difference between the number
of subjects responding "boy" versus "girl" on each of the critical items, a chi
square analysis was made of the raw data from each sub-sample. The results are
summarized in Figure 3.

The hypothesis under investigation was not disproved by the data obtained.
Figures 1 through 4 indicate that cultural expectations and sex role standards
were generally congruent in the samples studied in each country. The results also
support the proposition that cultural expectations and sex role standards differ
between countries.

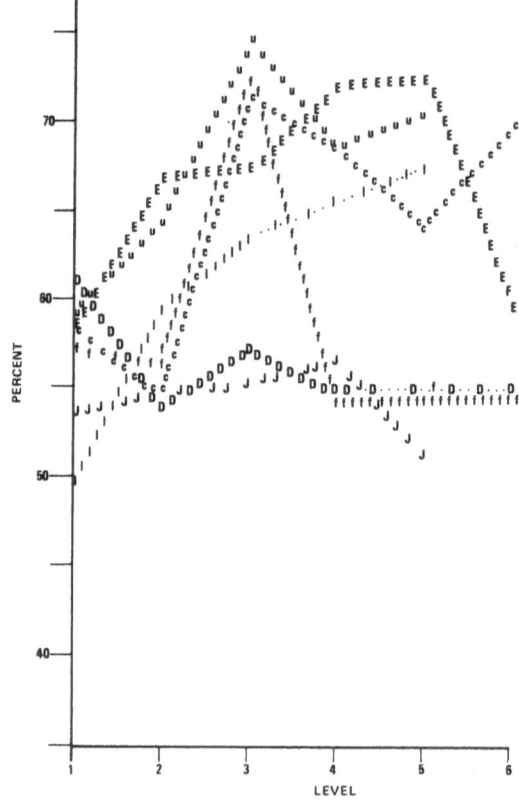

Fig. 1. Percent of female subjects responding "girl" at each level (items pooled). Letter indicates initial letter of name of country. Line with .. indicates intermediate level not tested.

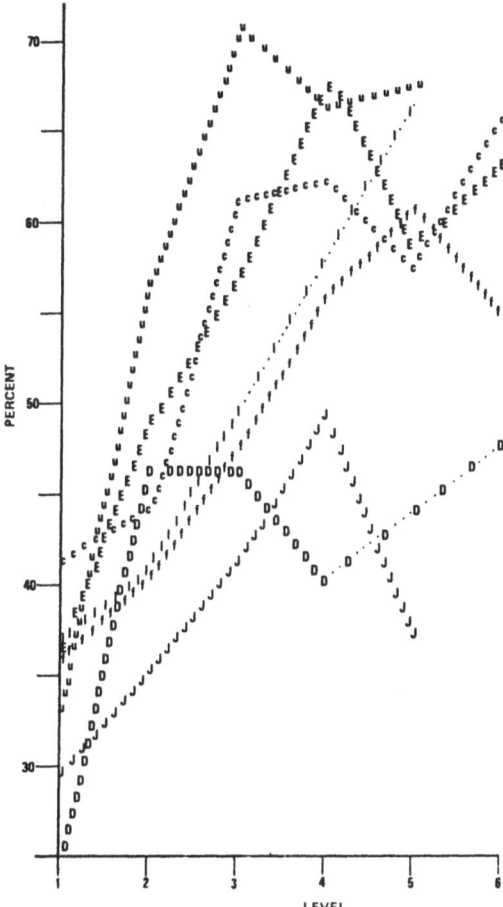

Fig. 2. Percent of male subjects responding "girl" at each level (items pooled). Letter indicates initial letter of name of country. Line with .. indicates intermediate level not tested.

TABLE I

Percent of female subjects' responses on all items that were "girl"

Country	Level											
	1		2		3		4		5		6	
	N	%	N	%	N	%	N	%	N	%	N	%
Canada	66	58.3	78	54.8	52	71.2	56	68.8	106	64.4	104	69.7
Denmark	42	60.1	38	53.9	28	57.1	15	55.0	*	*	166	55.3
England	45	58.3	46	66.8	50	67.5	33	72.0	95	72.6	49	59.2
Finland	61	57.4	66	56.4	48	72.4	67	54.1	64	54.3	96	54.4
Israel	48	49.5	48	59.4	50	63.5	*	*	50	67.5	*	*
Japan	37	53.4	33	54.5	38	55.3	34	56.6	54	51.4	*	*
U.S.A.	54	58.8	58	64.2	102	74.8	35	68.6	57	70.6	*	*

* indicates level was not tested

TABLE II
Percent of male subjects' responses on all items that were "girl"

Country	Level											
	1		2		3		4		5		6	
	N	%	N	%	N	%	N	%	N	%	N	%
Canada	64	42.2	74	44.3	34	61.1	43	62.2	45	57.8	97	65.5
Denmark	31	24.2	41	46.3	26	46.2	18	40.3	*	*	123	47.7
England	45	36.1	44	48.9	43	57.0	36	67.4	6	58.3	48	63.0
Finland	50	36.0	53	40.6	55	47.3	43	55.8	47	61.2	86	54.9
Israel	59	36.9	41	40.9	50	49.5	*	*	50	66.5	*	*
Japan	37	29.7	35	35.0	42	41.1	56	49.1	16	37.5	*	*
U.S.A.	71	33.1	70	56.4	100	70.5	42	66.7	16	67.2	*	*

* indicates level was not tested

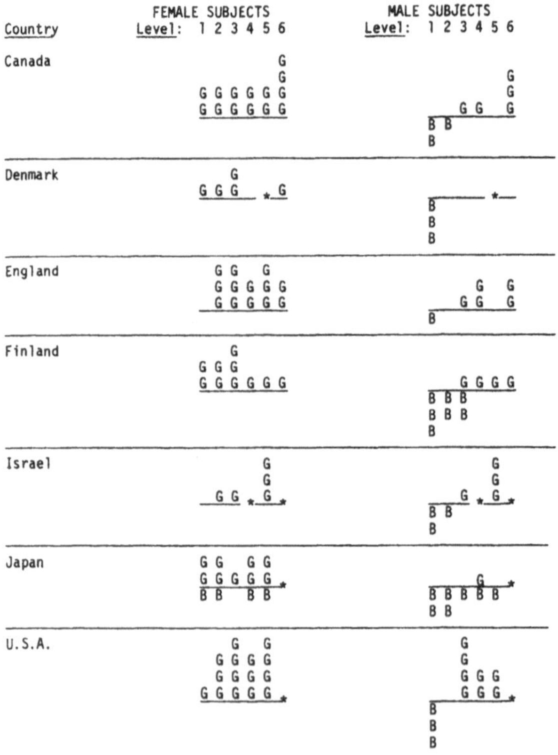

Fig. 3. Number of test items (out of 4) statistically significant (p < .05) on chi square analysis. 'G' indicates significantly more frequent response of 'girl'. 'B' indicates significantly more frequent response of 'boy'. '*' indicates level was not tested.

The attitudes in Denmark and Japan are especially divergent from the pattern found in the other five countries. This difference stands out more clearly in the responses of the male subjects than in those from the females. In Canada, England, Finland, Israel, and U.S.A. males begin by accepting reading as a masculine activity and then later switch to allocating it more to the feminine role, whereas in Japan and Denmark reading appears to be acceptable to males as a masculine activity at all age levels.

An experiment in Berlin, Germany using the same test materials obtained results similar to those reported above from Denmark and Japan. Reading was perceived by males of all ages as appropriate for the masculine role (Valtin, 1979).

These findings show at least that cultural attitudes toward reading as being suited more to one sex role than the other vary from country to country and that school children quite rapidly adopt these cultural values. The way in which sex role stereotypes may influence boys' and girls' accessibility to literacy is indicated by three studies.

Palardy (1969) reported that boy pupils whose first-grade teachers believed that boys are less successful than girls in learning to read, had poorer achievements in reading than a comparable group of boy pupils whose teachers believed that boys are as successful as girls in learning to read. Mazurkiewicz (1960) found that the reading achievement scores of a sample of eleventh-grade boys were higher for those students who considered reading as a masculine activity than for those students who perceived it as feminine. Dwyer's (1974) study of boys and girls in grades two to twelve revealed that sex role standards contributed significant variance to test scores in reading. She concluded that sex differences in reading "are more a function of the child's perception of these areas as sex-appropriate or sex-inappropriate than of the child's biological sex, individual preference for masculine or feminine sex-role, or liking or disliking of reading or arithmetic" (p. 811).

FUTURE ABROGATION OF INEQUITIES

In this paper I have discussed only published reports of educational, medical and psychological research on the differential treatment of boys and girls in regular schools and clinical situations. Most of such research has been conducted in North America, where, at the present time, it seems that for boys literacy is made less accessible in the regular education system but treatment for reading disability is more accessible than for girls. It is not suggested that there is a direct causal connection between these two phenomena. What is more probable is that they are both concomitants of the stereotype of reading as a feminine activity.

But, as our cross-national survey showed, sex role stereotypes about literacy behavior differ from country to country. Our survey was limited and it seems likely that in some other countries literacy may be regarded as more appropriate for males. For example, Abiri's large-scale reading experiment in Nigeria found that the Yoruba boys had superior achievements to those of the girls. This appeared to be related to the girls' comparatively poor school attendence. Downing and Thackray (1975) noted that in that part of Nigeria "if some chore needs doing around the homestead, the girl is kept at home to do it, while the boy is allowed to go to school" (p. 20). Wilks (1968) notes that the Muslim Dyula of Western Sudan "send many of their sons and some of their daughters to school" (p. 165). Oommen (1973) specifies another social attitude that makes literacy less accessible to girls in India: "Social causes are also an important factor in girls dropping out of school — betrothal, and the unwillingness of parents to send grown-up girls to a mixed school" (p. 410).

In conclusion, it is clear that inequities exist in the relative accessibility of literacy to females and males, and that social prejudices are at least in part responsible for them. Some societies discriminate against females. Others make literacy less readily available to males. It is a notoriously difficult task to change such social attitudes toward sex roles. Perhaps the greatest problem is that they are for the most part unconscious and therefore unrecognized. Hence, the first task that must be undertaken in these circumstances is that of helping people to become aware of the possibility that either boys or girls may be denied the fullest development of literacy skills through the unthinking perpetuation of customary sex role stereotypes. At the same time, educational organizations in countries such as the United States should consider using methods of demonstrating to the public that men can read as well as women and with equal enjoyment. In these countries, too, educators and clinicians should be alerted to the possibility that the diagnosis of dyslexia and reading disabilities in girls may be obstructed by lack of referral due to biassed expectancies among parents and teachers.

University of Victoria, Canada

REFERENCES

Abiri, J. O. O.
    1969 World Initial Teaching Alphabet Versus Traditional Orthography. Doctoral dissertation, University of Ibadan, Nigeria.
Alden, C. L., Sullivan, H. B., and Durrell, D. D.
    1941 The frequency of special reading disabilities. Education (Boston University) 62: 32–36.
Anderson, I. H., Hughes, B. O., and Dixon, W. R.
    1957 The rate of reading development and its relation to age of learning to read, sex, and intelligence. Journal of Educational Research 50: 481–494.
Blanchard, P.
    1936 Reading diabilities in relation to difficulties of personality and emotional development. Mental Hygiene 20: 384–413.
Carroll, M. W.
    1948 Sex differences in reading readiness at first grade level. Elementary English 25: 370–375.

Cobb, J. A., and Hops, H.
  1973 Effects of academic survival skill training on low achieving first graders. Journal of Educational Research 67: 108–113.
Critchley, M.
  1970 The Dyslexic Child. London: Heinemann.
Crosby, R. M. N.
  1969 Reading and the Dyslexic Child. London: Souvenir Press.
Downing, J., Dwyer, C. A. Feitelson, D., Jansen, M., Kemppainen, R., Matihaldi, H., Reggi, D. R., Sakamoto, T., Taylor, H., Thackray, D. V., and Thomson, D.
  1979 A cross-national survey of cultural expectations and sex role standards in reading. Journal of Research in Reading 2: 8–23.
Downing, J., and Thackray, D.
  1975 Reading Readiness. London: Hodder and Stoughton.
Downing, J., and Thomson, D.
  1977 Sex role stereotypes in learning to read. Research in the Teaching of English 11: 149–155.
Durrell, D. D.
  1940 Improvement of Basic Reading Abilities. Yonkers, N.Y.: World Book.
Dwyer, C. A.
  1973 Sex differences in reading. Review of Educational Research 43: 455–466.
Dwyer, C. A.
  1974 Influences of children's sex role standards on reading and arithmetic achievement. Journal of Educational Psychology 66: 811–816.
Dykstra, R., and Tinney, R.
  1969 Sex differences in reading readiness – first-grade achievement and second-grade achievement. In Figurel, J. A. (ed.), Reading and Realism. Newark, Del.: IRA.
Eisenberg, L.
  1966 The epidemiology of reading retardation and a program for preventive intervention. In Money, J. (ed.), The Disabled Reader. Baltimore, Maryland: Johns Hopkins Press.
Fernald, G. M.
  1943 Remedial Techniques in Basic School Subjects. New York: McGraw-Hill.
Gates, A. I.
  1961 Sex differences in reading ability. Journal of Educational Research 36: 594–603.
Goody, J.
  1968 Literacy in Traditional Societies. London: Cambridge University Press.
Gross, A. D.
  1978 Sex role standards and reading achievement: a study of an Israeli kibbutz system. Reading Teacher 32: 149–156.
Harris, A. J., and Sipay, E. R.
  1975 How to Increase Reading Ability. New York: David McKay.
Johnson, D. D.
  1973–1974 Sex differences in reading across cultures. Reading Research Quarterly 9: 67–68.
Kagan, J.
  1964 The child's sex role classification of school objects. Child Development 35: 1051–1056.
Konski, V.
  1955 An investigation into differences between boys and girls in selected reading readiness areas and in reading achievement. Reading Teacher, 8: 235–237.
Mazurkiewicz, A. J.
  1960 Social-cultural influences and reading. Journal of Developmental Reading 3: 254–263.

Miles, T. R.
   1974 The Dyslexic Child. London: Priory Press.
Ministry of Education
   1950 Reading Ability: Some Suggestions for Helping the Backward (pamphlet No. 18).
          London: her Majesty's Stationery Office.
Ministry of Education
   1957 Standards of Reading 1948 to 1956 (Pamphlet No. 32). London: Her Majesty's
          Stationery Office.
Monroe, M.
   1932 Children Who Cannot Read. Chicago: University of Chicago Press.
Morris, J. M.
   1966 Standard and Progress in Reading. Slough, England: National Foundation for
          Educational Research.
Oommen, C.
   1973 India. In Downing, J. (ed.), Comparative Reading. New York: Macmillan.
Orlow, M.
   1976 Literacy training in West Germany and the United States. Reading Teacher 29:
          460–467.
Palardy, J. M.
   1969 What teachers believe – what children achieve. Elementary School Journal 69:
          370–374.
Potter, M.
   1949 Perception of symbol orientation and early reading success. Contributions to
          Education, No 939. New York: Teachers' College, Columbia University.
Prescott, C. A.
   1955 Sex difference in Metropolitan readiness test results. Journal of Educational
          Research 48: 605–610.
Preston, R. C.
   1962 Reading achievement of German and American children. School and Society 90:
          350–354.
Pringle, M. L. K., Butler, N. R., and Davie, R.
   1966 11,000 Seven-Year-Olds. London: Longmans.
Samuels, F.
   1943 Sex differences in reading achievement. Journal of Educational Research 36:
          594–603.
Samuels, S. J., and Turnure, J. E.
   1974 Attention and reading achievement in first-grade boys and girls. Journal of Educa-
          tional Psychology 66: 29–32.
Schonell, F. J.
   1942 Backwardness in the Basic Subjects. Edinburgh: Oliver and Boyd.
Stein, A. H., and Smithells, J.
   1969 Age and sex differences in children's sex role standards about achievement.
          Developmental Psychology 1: 252–259.
Thackary, D. V.
   1965 A study of the relationship between some specific evidence of reading readiness
          and reading progress in the infant school. British Journal of Educational Psychol-
          ogy 35: 252–254.
Thackray, D. V.
   1971 Readiness to Read With i.t.a. and t.o. London: Geoffrey Chapman.
Valtin, R.
   1979 Personal communication.
Vernon, M. D.
   1957 Backwardness in Reading. London: Cambridge University Press.

Vittaniemi, E.
1965 Differences in reading between the sexes, I–II. Kasvatus ja Koulu (Education and School) 51: 122–131 and 173–180.
Wilks, I.
1968 The transmission of Islamic learning in the Western Sudan. In Goody, J. (ed.), Literacy in Traditional Societies. London: Cambridge University Press.
Young, R. A.
1938 Case studies in reading disability. American Journal of Orthopsychiatry 8: 230–254.

CATHLEEN A. BROWN, Ph.D.

SEX TYPING IN OCCUPATIONAL PREFERENCES OF HIGH SCHOOL BOYS AND GIRLS

THE PROBLEM

Each society establishes role descriptions of its women and its men, and within any given society there are expectations that members will develop according to the socially defined stereotypes. Through the process of socialization males and females acquire a set of beliefs, attitudes, and a range of behaviors which are consistent with the roles they are expected to play.

Families, schools, and social institutions provide cues through examples, expressed expectations, and reinforcement systems which influence sex role development. These social cues reinforce differences in the behavior of males and females, and these differences help perpetuate the traditional stereotypic beliefs about the abilities, personalities, preferences, and aspirations of men and women.

The sex role system as it functions in American society creates a difficult double bind for women. The role of wife and mother and the traditional feminine behaviors of nurturing, dependence, passivity, and submissiveness are not valued by our society. Value is placed on productivity, profits, and achievement in careers. Recognition goes to those who succeed in the marketplace of occupational skills.

Women are caught in a conflict. If they conform to the role prescribed, they are excluded from opportunities to share in the valued occupational activities and their behavior is termed unhealthy for adults by mental health clinicians (Broverman, et al., 1972). If they defy convention, they risk alienation and doubts about their femininity (Bardwick, 1971; Maccoby, 1963).

The restrictions which the traditional role places on females has become widely recognized in recent years. Values are internalized by both sexes nonconsciously and the limitations which these place upon individuals is often accepted as normal and irrefutable (Bem and Bem, 1970). Unless nonconscious stereotypical beliefs are brought into conscious awareness, the likelihood of their changing is very remote. It is difficult to effect changes in belief systems unless those beliefs are available to the conscious thought processes.

A major goal of those responsible for the education and healthy development of children should be to bring nonconscious sex role beliefs into conscious awareness. This could free both males and females from the limitations of the stereotyped roles and enable them to select occupational goals as an expression of their individual interests and abilities.

The aim of this paper is to gain greater understanding of sex typing of occupations by exploring the career preferences of high school students. A brief review

81

I. Gross, J. Downing, and A. d'Heurle (eds.), Sex Role Attitudes and Cultural Change, 81–88.
Copyright © 1982 by D. Reidel Publishing Company.

of occupational patterns is given as background to the students' aspirations, and a review of studies which have examined sex typing in career choices of young children is included.

OCCUPATIONAL PATTERNS OF WOMEN WORKERS

More than 50 percent of all women ages 18 to 64 are working, and nine out of ten girls will work some time in their lives. Despite an ever increasing number of women workers the occupational sex typing has persisted virtually unchanged throughout the twentieth century (Gross, 1968; Oppenheimer, 1970; U.S. Department of Labor, 1975). Although a small number of women have entered traditionally masculine fields, the large majority of women are still confined to traditional women's occupations. Nearly half of all women workers are employed in ten occupations: secretary, retail sales, bookkeepers, private household workers, elementary school teaching, typist, cashier, stitchers, sewing, and nursing.

The majority of women are employed in highly sex-segregated, low paying jobs that require little if any on-the-job training. Such jobs are of low status, rarely challenge the intellectual resources of the individual, and tend to be easy to enter and exit. The jobs that most women hold are in themselves barriers to further advancement because they often lack opportunities for promotion and consequently carry little incentive for further training or diversity of experience.

Gains have been made in the number of women employed in the professions, but they are abysmally small. The number of women lawyers has grown from 2.4 percent in 1960 to 4.7 percent in 1973. The number of physicians has grown from 7 percent in 1960 to 9 percent in 1973, while women dentists have grown from 2.3 percent in 1960 to 3.4 percent in 1973 (U.S. Department of Labor, 1975).

Income is another measure which reflects occupational limitations on women. In 1973 women who worked full time earned an average of 57 percent of what men earned (Dixon, 1975). This figure reflects a decrease of 1 percent since incomes were first reported in 1939. Income differences between men and women doing the same work are continuing to widen (Trieman and Terrell, 1975). Despite efforts of the women's movement and federal and state legislation, sex typing in careers continues to limit women to low paying, less challenging, and low status occupational positions.

RESEARCH ON SEX TYPING IN CAREER CHOICES OF
YOUNG CHILDREN

Understanding the way in which sex role socialization takes place has been the focus of many recent studies. Several researchers have attempted to learn at what age sex role typing of careers becomes evident. Wirtenberg (1976) suggests that traditional educational institutions have contributed to occupational stratification by sex through textbooks and instructional materials, differential curricula for boys and girls, and through discrimination in vocational counseling. It is difficult to attribute more than a portion of the blame to schools, however, because studies are finding that sex typing is evident in the earliest school years.

Looft (1971) found that first and second grade boys named more than twice as many occupations as girls when asked, "What do you want to be when you grow up?" More than three-fourths of the girls named either nurse or teacher as their first choice. Several girls said they would be mothers, whereas not one boy said he would be a father. Girls apparently use their mothers as role models and choose to do what their mothers do, while boys apparently recognize that their fathers are defined by what they do outside the home, rather than within it.

In a study of 9 through 17 year olds Barnett (1973) found that girls of all ages choose lower ranking occupations than boys. This supports the findings of Bem and Bem (1970) which showed that by ninth grade 25 percent of the boys chose science or engineering while only 3 percent of the girls did.

From the earliest grades girls show restrictions in the range of occupations open to them. By the time formal education is completed, there are gross differences in the expectations, aspirations, and preparation that men and women have for careers. Understanding the extent of sex typing is essential to developing effective programs to change these patterns. The purpose of this study is to gain information about sex typing as it is expressed in the career preferences of high school girls and boys.

THE STUDY

Subjects in the study were 308 students in grades 7 through 12 who volunteered to participate. The students attended two junior high schools and two senior high schools, and resided in middle income neighborhoods of three suburban cities located forty-five minutes from a major metropolitan city. Subjects were given a careers survey by their teachers in class. The author administered the survey in two classes and videotaped class discussions following completion of the surveys. The survey was developed by the author to measure the extent of sex typing and to assess the influence of parents' occupations and role models' occupations on the subjects' choices.

Subjects were asked to list five choices of careers they thought they would like, and to number them in order of preference from 1 through 5. They were then asked, "If you were of the opposite sex, what five careers do you think you would like?" They were asked to rank order these five choices also. Subjects were asked to list the occupations of their mothers, fathers, and a role model (think of a person you know who works at something you might like to do).

CAREERS SURVEY

1. Mark your age group.

   8-12 years_____ 13-18 years_____ 19-24 years_____ over 24_____

2. Mark your sex. M_____ F_____

3. Grade_____ School _____

4. List five careers you think you would like.

   _____   _____

   _____   _____

   _____   _____

   _____   _____

   _____   _____

5. Put a #1 beside the one you like best, a #2 beside one you like next, and a #3 beside the next, and so on.

6. If you were of the opposite sex, what five careers do you think you would like?

   _____   _____

   _____   _____

   _____   _____

   _____   _____

   _____   _____

7. Put a #1 beside the one you like best and so on.

8. Think of a person you know who works at something you might like to do. What does that person do?

   _____

9. What kind of work does your father do?

   _____

10. What kind of work does your mother do?

   _____

Cathleen A. Brown
414 Yale Avenue
Claremont, California   Copyright 1977

To analyze the data the career choices were categorized using a system based on the Department of Labor's Categories of Occupations. The categories were ranked on levels of professionalism determined by the academic preparation and training required for the occupation. The category of professional workers which included doctors, dentists, scientists, engineers, artists, and writers, and college teachers was given the rank of one, while service workers, housewives, and unemployed were ranked fifteen, sixteen, and eighteen. Categories were labeled to indicate whether they were dominated by male workers, or by female workers. If 70 percent of the workers in a category were of one sex it was labeled as dominated by that sex. If neither sex had more than 70 percent workers in the category, it was labeled as a category with an equal number of men and women. The categories, their rankings, and their labels are listed below.

1.   Professional workers (male 75%)
2.   Secondary teachers (equal)
3.   Elementary teachers (female 84%)
4.   Technical workers, lab technicians, librarians, accountants (male 75%)
5.   Nurses (female 82%)
6.   Managers and administrators (male 81%)
7.   Self employed business (male 95%)
8.   Self employed, models and actresses (female)
9.   Sales (equal)
10.   Clerical workers (female 77%)
11.   Crafts (male 96%)
12.   Operatives (equal)
13.   Farmers (male 85%)
14.   Service, foods, health care (female 75%)
15.   Service, mail carriers, janitors (male 74%)
16.   Housewives (female)
17.   Military service (male)
18.   Unemployed
19.   Bizarre responses

RESULTS

The results show that sex typing in careers is evident in the preferences expressed by these high school students. (Significance was determined by t tests with a p value of .05 or smaller.) Girls chose significantly less professional occupations for themselves than they chose as if they were boys. Males chose significantly more professional careers for themselves than they chose as if they were girls. Seven girls out of the total of 170 (4%) chose the same occupations for themselves and for the opposite sex. Three boys out of the total of 138 (2%) chose the same occupations for both sexes. These small percentages indicate that very few of the subjects were free of stereotyped expectations. Ninety-four percent of the girls and 98 percent of the boys changed their choices when the sex of the responder changed.

Nonconscious values appear to determine occupational choices. However, when discussions followed the completion of the surveys, students began to show awareness of these nonconscious beliefs.

"If I were a boy, I would be a mechanic."

"You can be a mechanic if you want to."

"Yeah, my brother's girlfriend helps him fix his car."

"Boys can't be cooks."

"Oh yes they can. I know, because my father does the cooking."

When nonconscious attitudes are expressed, they immediately touch the conscious awareness of others, and reaction against the stereotype emerges rapidly. The members of this particular discussion group ended by concluding there were no jobs which girls or boys could not do if they chose to.

There appears to be a greater degree of stereotyping about the opposite sex than there is about one's own sex. There was no significant difference in the level of professionalism of the occupations selected by girls for themselves and by boys for themselves. However, when girls chose occupations as if they were boys, they chose significantly more professional occupations than boys chose for themselves. Boys also showed this stereotyped response by choosing significantly less professional occupations for the opposite sex than girls chose for themselves. The sexes appear to have rigid views of one another. They project onto the other sex an even greater degree of stereotyped thinking than they exhibit for their own sex. The sexes are more alike than they imagine. One focus of a program to bring about change would have to deal with females' notions about males' notions about females.

The influence from fathers, mothers, and role models was measured by counting the number of occupations a subject listed which showed a marked similarity to the occupations of father, mother, or role model. For example, if a father's occupation was listed as construction worker and the subject chose carpenter as an occupation, it would be scored as influenced by his father's occupation.

Role models influenced both girls and boys choices more than either parents' occupations. Almost half of the girls (49%), and 43 percent of the boys showed some influence from the role models' occupation. Nineteen percent of the boys, but only 4 percent of the girls had a choice which was influenced by the father's occupation. Mothers' occupations influenced 12 percent of the girls' choices, but only 4 percent of the boys.

The impact of role models on both girls and boys suggests this would be an effective means of changing career stereotyping. Contacts with role models in non-traditional careers could help break the stereotyped thinking which limits career choices. Since adolescence is a time when young people normally move away from parental influence and toward non-family attachments, it is an appropriate time to utilize the impact of role models. Contacts between role models and adolescents should be an integral part of career education programs.

A curious fact emerged from the data. Nineteen of the boys did not answer the section based on opposite sex responses. They did, however, proceed on to complete the parental and role model occupations. The meaning of their avoidance of this section is unclear. Is the perception of the world "as if one were female" too threatening for some to respond to? What causes this? This question would be interesting to pursue, and possibly has some bearing on the problems of sex role definitions.

CONCLUSIONS

Sex typing in careers persists in the career choices of high school boys and girls, and nonconscious beliefs affect the responses. The stereotyping of the opposite sex shows more extreme attitudes than does the thinking about one's own sex. Girls expect boys will have more professional careers than boys choose for themselves, and boys expect girls to have less professional careers than girls choose to have. Programs aimed at changing stereotyped beliefs should closely attend to the expectations and attitudes which members of each sex have about the other. Verbal expression of nonconscious beliefs brings them into awareness and precipitates a conscious decision about changing or retaining the belief. This appears to be an effective way to eliminate stereotypes.

The strong influence of role models on the choices of both boys and girls suggest that role models could be used effectively to change the traditional patterns of thinking. Career education programs should include role models as an integral part of the curriculum.

Recent legislation and social movements aimed at equal opportunities for women do not appear to affect stereotyping of careers. This suggests that a large part of the responsibility for changing sex typing in career preferences will fall to educators and mental health professionals. Full equality of access to occupational opportunities can only be achieved by the active commitment and effort of educators and professionals concerned about the healthy development of all males and females.

BIBLIOGRAPHY

Barnett, R.
    1973 Vicissitudes of occupational preferences and aversion among boys and girls age 9–17. Paper presented at American Psychological Association, Montreal, August.
Bem, D. and Bem, S.
    1970 We're all nonconscious sexists. In D. J. Bem (ed.), Beliefs, Attitudes, and Human Affairs. Monterey, CA: Wadsworth.
Bem, S. D. and Bem, D. J.
    1970 Case study of a nonconscious ideology: Training the woman to know her place. In D. J. Bem (ed.), Beliefs, Attitudes, and Human Affairs. Belmont, Calif.: Brooks/ Cole.
Broverman, I. K., Vogel, S. R., Broverman, D. M., Clarkson, F. E., and Rosenkrantz, P. S.
    1972 Sex role stereotypes: A current appraisal. Journal of Social Issues 38(2): 59– 78.

Dixon, Ruth B.
   1976 Measuring equality between the sexes. Journal of Social Issues 32(3): 19–32.
Duncan, B. and Evers, M.
   1975 Measuring change in attitudes toward women's work. In R. C. Land and S.
           Spilerman (eds.), Social Indicator Models. New York: Russell Sage.
Dweck, C. S.
   1975 Sex differences in the meaning of negative evolution in achievement situations:
           Determinants and consequences. Paper presented at Society for Research in
           Child Development, Denver.
Farmer, Helen S. and Thomas, E. Backer
           Women at work: 'Things are looking up.' Report prepared by Human Interaction
           Institute, Los Angeles, California.
Gross, E.
   1968 Plus ça change: The sexual structure of occupations over time. Social Problems
           (Fall): 198–208.
Keller, S.
   1973 The future role of women. Annals of the American Academy of Political and
           Social Science 408: 1–12.
Kohlberg, L. A.
   1966 A cognitive-developmental analysis of children's sex role concepts and attitudes.
           In E. E. Maccoby (ed.), The Development of Sex Differences. Stanford, CA:
           Stanford University Press.
Lipman-Blumen, J.
   1972 How ideology shapes women's lives. Scientific American 226: 34–42.
Looft, W. R.
   1971 Sex differences in the expression of vocational aspirations by elementary school
           children. Developmental Psychology 5: 366.
Oppenheimer, V. K.
   1970 The female labor force in the United States. Population Monographs, Series #5,
           Berkeley, CA: Institute of International Studies.
Parsons, J. E., Frieze, I. H., Ruble, D. N., and Croke, J.
   1975 Intropsychic factors influencing career aspirations in college women. Unpublished
           manuscript.
Stevenson, M.
   1973 Women's wages and job segregation. Politics and Society: 83–96.
Tangri, Sandra
   1972 Determinants of occupational role innovation among college women. Journal
           of Social Issues 28(2): 177–200.
Trieman, D. J., and Terrell, K.
   1975 Women, work, and wages: Trends in the female occupation structure In K. C.
           Lana and S. Spilerman (eds.) Social Indicator Models. New York: Russell Sage.
U.S. Department of Labor
   1972 Handbook on Women Workers. Women's Bureau Bulletin. Washington, D. C.: U.S.
           Government Printing Office.
U.S. Department of Labor
   1975 Handbook on Women Workers, Bulletin 297.
Wirtenberg, T. H., and Nakamura, C. T.
   1976 Education: Barrier or boon to changing occupational roles of women? Journal
           of Social Issues 32(3): 165–179.
Zellman, Gail
   1976 The role of structural factors in limiting women's institutional participation.
           Journal of Social Issues 32(3): 33–46.

†CORINNE HUTT, Ph.D.

ASPIRATIONS AND SEX ROLES – ARE THEY IN CONFLICT?

The underachievement of girls, at all levels of ability, is now well documented. The recent EEC report attributes this underachievement to "discrimination and sex-stereotyping". Discrimination there occasionally may be, but sex-stereotyping is a facile term too often used to stifle inquiry rather than stimulate it. Are girls reluctant to go into tertiary education because they construe it as masculine? Or are girls making a decision based on a realistic assessment of their prospective role conflicts?

In a pilot study, we sought to identify some of the attitudes of boys and girls towards academic subjects, towards jobs, towards competition with the opposite sex and towards achievement. Another objective of the study was to examine how these attitudes differed between pupils in single-sex and those in mixed-sex schools. Preliminary results suggest that stereotyping of academic subjects and jobs is far less evident than the reluctance to compete, particularly amongst the girls. It may be recalled that Dale (1974) found that the achievement of boys in mixed-sex schools was far greater than that of boys' schools, even though the latter schools had the advantage in overall ability, socio-economic background, good teaching etc. Thus, the most likely explanation for this superior performance is that boys respond favourably to the challenge of competition with girls. Girls however, do not appear to respond so well to competition and in many respects their performance is better in a girls' only school. Thus the 'stereotyping' of roles is an oversimplification of the processes at work.

In the development of sex roles there are many factors that operate upon the individual and social group. Some germane factors in these broad contexts are considered so that the conflicts inherent in the articulation and realisation of these roles may be examined.

First, sex role differentiation in childhood may be conceived of as an epigenetic process (Hutt, 1978), in which perceptual and behavioural propensities, parental expectations, imitation and identification, and the influence of the media all play a part. In many ways a child's propensities and parental expectations often accord well with each other, as when parents manifest a preference for interaction with same-sex child (Weinraub and Frankel, 1978) or when mothers talk more to their infant daughters who are both more responsive to their mother's speech and vocalise more (Kagan 1969; McGuiness, 1975). The influence of the media on the other hand produces a discordant note: both in children's literature and in children's TV the female is portrayed as insipid, insignificant or inconspicuous (Weitzman et al., 1972; Sternglanz and Serbin, 1974; Tavris and Offir, 1977). Paradoxically however, early social pressures permit a greater variety of behaviours and more flexibility in the female role

89

I. Gross, J. Downing, and A. d'Heurle (eds.), Sex Role Attitudes and Cultural Change, 89–91.
Copyright © 1982 by D. Reidel Publishing Company.

while boys are constrained to adopt appropriate sex role behaviours earlier and more strongly than girls. How do children reconcile these paradoxes, or do we accept the sardonic comment of Sternglanz and Serbin: "female children are taught that almost the only way to be a successful human being if you are female is through the use of magic"?

Secondly, in later childhood, parental and social expectations become more prescriptive, and approval of peers more important, with the consequence that nonconformity to stereotype becomes more difficult. At this age however, the conflicts for girls are far worse than they are for boys. Implicit in the educational system is the assumption that each individual will strive to fulfil his/her potential. But this involves competition with the opposite sex which girls dislike more than boys. Boys are defensive in relation to bright girls – thus girls feel constrained to minimise the extent of their ability. Alternatively, certain subjects are characterised by the performance of one sex more than the other – for instance, maths and science are subjects at which boys are better, languages and biology are those at which girls do better, as a result, girls are reluctant to opt for the more prestigious, 'masculine' subjects, and continue to choose the traditional, non-career options. Their aspirations are severely limited by personal and social constraints.

Thirdly, in adolescence and early adult life, the ambitions and achievements of women are often curtailed by the demands of their feminine and domestic roles. Marriage and a family limit a woman's achievement and there is difficulty in justifying persistent endeavour and expense in pursuit of a career that is more than likely to be interrupted. Thus, girls and women experience conflicts between their aspirations and the realisation of the feminine role, conflicts which are seldom experienced by men.

In the development of feminine and masculine roles, therefore, there is an asymmetry which is seldom acknowledged. The dissonance between a girl's aptitudes and aspirations on the one hand and social expectation on the other, are far greater than they ever are for a boy. Boys too may experience such dissonance if they wish to take up traditionally 'feminine' careers like nursing or midwifery, but it is less pervasive. The sources of conflict in the development of sex roles need to be identified before we can understand how a healthy reconciliation may be forged.

University of Keele

† deceased

REFERENCES

Dale, R. R.
    1974 Mixed or Single-Sex School: Attainment, Attitudes and Overview. Vol. 3. London: Routledge & Kegan Paul.
Hutt, C.
    1978 Sex role differentiation in social development. In: McGurk, H. (ed.), Issues in Childhood Social Development. London: Methuen.

Kagan, J.
   1969 On the meaning of behaviour: illustrations from the infant. Child Development
        40: 1121–34.
McGuiness, D.
   1975 Away from a unisex psychology: individual differences in visual sensory and
        perceptual processes. Perception 6: 22–32.
Sternglanz, S. H. and Serbin, L. A.
   1974 Sex role stereotypes in children's television programmes. Development Psychology
        10: 710–15.
Tavris, C. and Offir, C.
   1977 The Longest War: Sex Differences in Perspective. New York: Harcourt Brace
        Jovanovich Inc.
Weinraub, M. and Frankel, J.
   1978 Sex differences in parent-infant interaction during free play, departure and
        separation. Child Development.
Weitzman, L. J. Eifler, D., Hokada, E. and Ross, C.
   1972 Sex role socialization in picture books for preschool children. American Journal
        of Sociology 77: 1125–50.

ADMA D'HEURLE, Ph.D., JEFFREY COHEN, Ph.D., and
V. WIDMARK-PETERSSON, M.A.

CROSS-SEX FRIENDSHIP IN THE ELEMENTARY SCHOOL

SUMMARY. A survey of the presence of the theme of friendship in a sample of American and Swedish fourth and fifth grade readers was made. The results indicated that the theme of friendship in general and cross-sex friendship in particular appeared in only a small number of the stories. Sociometric questions given to fifth grade children showed that the majority of choices for instrumental and affective experiences went to same sex peers. This preliminary study indicates that in these two aspects of the elementary school culture cross-sex friendship is not indicated as a positive value.

INTRODUCTION

The importance of the school as an agent in the socialization of children in general and a force in determining sex role attitudes in particular has been widely recognized. Educational research has in recent years sought to determine the degree to which the school is able to affect change in the value system — the accepted wisdom of the cultural tradition that it represents. Research has also sought to establish the relative importance of the different means by which the school maintains and perpetuates a particular value system or worldview; its educational materials, the methods of instruction, the school's organization, its style of management and its hidden curriculum, the intangible but real quality of its intellectual and social climate — its particular cultural pattern.

The present study is an extension of this boy of research that underscores the role of the school in socialization and its effect on developing sex role expectations, standards and attitudes (Downing, 1979). The study aims specifically to explore the influence of the school on the development of cross-sex friendship among elementary school children by examining (1) the treatment of the theme in the current upper-elementary school readers in two Western societies — the U.S. and Sweden, and (2) children's own account of their friendships with school peers of the same or opposite sex.

Underlying this hypothesis-generating, preliminary exploration of the theme of cross-sex friendship are the assumptions that (1) the psychological study of friendship has been woefully neglected, (2) cross-sex peer friendship in childhood is an important means for the development of healthy sex role attitudes and (3) reading materials are a potential source of role models and expectations that could affect children's developing and changing attitudes.

Although friendship is generally considered a positive value like motherhood and patriotism, it has become as C. S. Lewis (1960) has so convincingly argued, one of the least meaningful forms of love in modern times. This view has more recently found strong support in cross-cultural research. Brain (1976), for example, has demonstrated how friendship is given a central place in many traditional societies and how it is strengthened by formal bonds and bolstered by revered

93

I. Gross, J. Downing, and A. d'Heurle (eds.), Sex Role Attitudes and Cultural Change, 93–100.
Copyright © 1982 by D. Reidel Publishing Company.

social institutions. He maintains that almost by definition Western Christian democratic forms of social accommodations imply the attenuation of friendship.

Many currents in the Western tradition have been indicated as possible causes for the current status of friendship and its marginal position in social scientific research. Among these currents are the unique stress on romantic love, the prevailing ambivalence towards homosexuality and the increased preoccupation with eroticism. Beyond these general cultural trends, modern psychological research, focused as it has been on parent-child interaction in early childhood, and the development of heterosexual behavior and of ego identity in adolescence, has tended to by-pass the period mistakenly named latency and the peer relations of boys and girls of this age group.

For the purposes of this study we have adopted a general definition of friendship and sought to circumscribe it roughly in a manner that is indicated in the salient social-science literature. Friendship, according to the classical definition of George Simmel, is a relationship that is built "at least in its idea upon the person in its totality". Because it lacks the vehemence of love and its frequent unevenness, friendship, Simmel stresses, "is more apt than love to connect a whole person with another" (Wolff, 1974: 325). Simmel's perceptive analysis touches upon the difficulties that the modern differentiated ego faces in entering such total relationships and concludes that , except for young children who are capable or total ego investment, the modern way of feeling tends more heavily toward differentiated friendships (Wolff, 1974: 326). Brain stresses the quality of equality between friends. "Even in lopsided relations between a patron and a client", he writes, "the use of the term 'friend' at least implies an attempt to equalize the relationship drawing persons of different status towards each other" (Brain, 1976: 20). Reciprocity, cooperation and complementarity have also been indicated as characteristics of friendship or at least, its matrix (Brain, 1976, 1977; Brenton, 1975; Peevers and Secord, 1973; Lewis, 1960). In their studies of primary groups and adult cross-sex friendship, Bates and Babchuk (1961) and Booth and Hess (1974) point to an affective dimension in addition to the cognitive-behavioral elements reflected in 'reciprocity', 'cooperation' and 'common interests'. This element of positive affect is manifest in the friends' mutual liking, trust, expressions of concern and the felt freedom to make demands on one another. The two dimensions are suggestive of Talcott Parsons' expressive and instrumental determinants (Parsons, 1954).

In our review of the contents of the school readers, we sought to make judgements regarding the presence or absence of friendship themes congruent with the view of friendship gleened from the above references. The same was true of the specific questions that we put to the children regarding their actual friendships.

METHOD

Part I

Nine American and seven Swedish school readers were used in this survey. The criteria for selection were that the books be officially defined as fourth and fifth grade readers that are currently and widely used in the public schools of both countries. Each book was read by one of the authors and a tally was made of the number of times that the theme of friendship was mentioned. The results for the American texts are presented in Table I and for the Swedish texts in Table II.

Part II

Two sociometric questions inviting the choice of peers to help with school related work or share a secret were used. (For exact text of questions see Appendix III). The subjects consisted of all available members of a fifth grade in a suburban public school. One hundred and thirteen children participated (56 boys and 57 girls). One child only chose not to make any choice.

In his presentation of the task to the subjects the experimenter stressed that it was not a test. He introduced the study briefly describing it as an effort to learn more about children's friendships. The subjects were asked to give their grade and gender and the first names of the three peers that they choose. Where the first name was unclear as to gender the subjects were asked to specify. The experimenter then read the questions aloud while the students read them silently before their choices were made. The results are presented in Table III and Table IV.

RESULTS

TABLE I
Friendship themes
American Texts

| | Child | | | Child-Adult | | | | Adult | | | |
	B–B	G–G	B–G	B–M	B–W	G–M	G–W	M–M	W–W	W–M	Total
number	18	8	9	11	4	4	1	5	5	2	64
percentage	3.3%	1.5%	1.7%	2.1%	.75%	.75%	.18%	.93%	.37%	.37%	11.8%

number of texts = 9
number of units = 540

TABLE II
Friendship themes
Swedish Texts

| | Child | | | Child-Adult | | | | Adult | | | |
	B–B	G–G	B–G	B–M	B–W	G–M	G–W	M–M	W–W	W–M	Total
number	9	4	4	1	0	2	0	0	0	0	20
percentage	2.8%	1.2%	1.2%	.31%		.61%					6.2%

number of texts = 7
number of units = 324

An examination of Table I and II shows that the theme of friendship appeared relatively infrequently in both the American and Swedish readers. Only 11.8 percent of the discrete units in the American books and 6.2 percent in the Swedish books, whatever their subject matter, mentioned friendship at all. The mention of cross-sex friendship between children was also quite rare and between adult men and women rarer still.

The findings from the Swedish texts did not confirm our expectations that the theme of cross-sex friendship would be more salient. Various qualitative differences between the thematic contents of the American and the Swedish texts were noted but these differences did not relate to the treatment of the theme of friendship in general and or cross-sex friendship in particular.

A slight tendency is noted for male friendships to be depicted more often than the other types. This tendency is more marked in the American readers.

TABLE III
Same and Cross-Sex Sociometric Choices

	Instrumental (Homework)		Expressive (Secret)	
Boys				
N = 56	B	G	B	G
possible R's = 168	145	19	148	10
	86.3%	11.3%	88.1%	6.0%
Girls				
N = 57	B	G	B	G
possible R's = 171	3	166	1	166
	1.8%	97.1%	.6%	97.1%

Note: Not all students gave 3 responses thus percentages do not total to 100%.

TABLE IV
Number of Children Crossing Gender Lines in 1 or more of their choices

	Instrumental	Expressive
Boys		
N = 56	N = 19	N = 10
	34%	17.9%
Girls		
N = 57	N = 3	N = 1
	5.3%	1.8%

Table III and IV present a summary of the sociometric data. The striking finding here is that children's choices of peers to share a secret or to help with work-related tasks are predominantly restricted to members of the chooser's own sex. A tendency for boys to cross the gender line on both questions is of interest and could be given different interpretations. This tendency may be viewed as a mark of confidence in their masculine role and evidence of general psychological maturity on the part of the boys who directed choices to girls. It could also represent continued dependence on competent and trustworthy female figures. Regrettably, our data does not provide a means for evaluating the motives under-lying the subject's sociometric choice. We must also stress the fact that whenever choices crossed gender lines, they invariably represented only one of the three choices made. Furthermore, it was noted that when boys and girls crossed gender lines they were more willing to cross for an instrumental task. Obviously, it is less threatening to share schoolwork with a member of the other sex than a secret.

Although not directly relevant to the central questions raised in this study, we include here a brief list of our impressionistic comparisons of the American and Swedish readers:

(1) A marked tendency was noted in the Swedish books to contain fewer stories that fall in what oculd be identified as a genre of psychosocial realism. In comparison to the American books, they included more legends, folktales and literary short stories by known modern authors.

(2) The contents of the Swedish texts appeared by American standards to be more appropriately geared for younger children. It is unclear whether this represents lower performance norms or a simple difference in the relative impor-tance ascribed to childrens' literature.

(3) Although the Swedish texts did not contain as many stories relating to daily social realities, they tended to select more serious social problems and deal with them more realistically.

(4) Sports were a less prominent theme in the Swedish texts. There was also a deemphasis on winning. Children appeared less often as successful achievers deserving of rewards and were more often in positions that required assurance and guidance from the adults.

DISCUSSION

Our survey of a sample of educational materials and the childrens' statements about their social relationships within the school lead us to conclude that the contemporary school continues to be primarily a conveyer of the prevalent value system. We do not suggest a causal relation between the absence of models of cross-sex friendships in the school books and the childrens' tendency to confine their close interpersonal relations to members of their own sex. However, we see both phenomena as expressions of a cultural ethos that, in its devaluation of cross-sex friendship, contributes to the conventional identification of things masculine and feminine, the resultant arbitrary delineation of spheres of interest, achievement and concern, and ultimately to the restriction of male and female interaction to erotic or romantic relations.

The meaning of friendship in human experience in general and particularly cross-sex friendship at different stages of development is due for serious re-evaluation by psychologists and educators. The time has come to put in proper perspective the psychological theories of Sullivan (1940) and Erikson (1950) which have been used to legitimize the stress on gender-binding and the devaluation of cross-sex friendship in the preadolescent years.

Historically, Sullivan's emphasis on peer relations in preadolescence was of great value in directing attention to a stage of development that had at the time that he was writing, received scant attention. Much in Sullivan's view of development is of incomparable value. However, there is in his emphasis on the homosexual quality of preadolescent friendship an element of bias that can be understood in the context of his total approach.

A close reading of Erikson suggests that he intended the stress to rest on the quality of reciprocity and cooperation in peer relations. His mention of the fact that close ties at this age are often between members of the same sex is more of a descriptive statement that is incidental to his emphasis on the quality of the relationship.

Faithfulness to the spirit of Sullivan and Erikson requires the continued reevaluation of aspects of development at the various stages of the life cycle in the light of knowledge about the biological organism and the social context. Contemporary scholarship dealing with the meaning of sexuality from psycho-historical and cross-cultural perspectives (Foucault, 1978, Rosaldo, 1974), the vast body of research on the psychology of sex differences (Maccoby and Jacklin, 1974) and sex role socialization (Katz, 1977; Money, 1972; Spence, 1978; Weitz, 1977) have shed new light on the developmental tasks of the juvenile period. The restriction of the child's close relations to same-age peers appears to be more a function of the dominant cultural ideology than a universal requirement of a critical period in the developmental process.

The efforts that have been made so far in examining the sexist bias in the elementary school curriculum and in the school educational practices and organizational arrangements (Guttentag and Bray, 1976; Weizman and Rizzo, 1974) are a first step in making explicit the unstated assumptions and the implied values that are sustained through the various parameters of the school culture. To undertake to encourage a broad range of interactions among boys and girls in the school and to seek purposefully to cultivate cross-sex friendships will require more positive action on behalf of educators. This is undoubtedly a difficult step considering the many demands that are being made of the school in the modern technological society. Its undertaking will depend on the answer that will be given to Counts' question of many decades ago (1932) *Dare the Schools Build a New Social Order?*

Mercy College, Dobbs Ferry, N.Y. (A. d'H.)
Ardsley Public Schools, Ardsley on Hudson, N.Y. (J. C.)
Nursing College, Uppsala (V. W.-P.)

REFERENCES

Bates, Alan P. and Babchuk, N.
    1961 The primary group: a reappraisal. Sociological Quarterly 2: 181–191.
Booth, A. and Hess, E.
    1974 Cross-sex friendship. Journal of Marriage and the Family: 38–47.
Brain, R.
    1976 Friends and Lovers. London: Granada Publishing.
Brain, R.
    1977 Somebody else should be your own best friend. Psychology Today: 83–126.
Brenton, M.
    1975 Friendship. New York: Stein and Day.
Counts, G.
    1932 Dare the School Build a New Social Order. John Day Company.
Downing, J.
    (Unpublished manuscript). Making literacy equally accessible to female and males.
Erikson, E.
    1950 Childhood and Society. New York: W. W. Norton.
Foucault, Michel
    1978 The History of Sexuality. New York: Pantheon Books.
Guttentag, M. and Bray, H.
    1976 Undoing Sex Stereotypes. New York: McGraw Hill.
Katz, L. et al.
    1977 Sex Role Socialization in Early Childhood. ERIC Document No. 148 472.
Lewis, C. S.
    1960 The Four Loves. New York: Harcourt Brace Jovanovich, pp. 106–107, 82–127.
Maccoby, E. E. and Jacklin, C. N.
    1974 The Psychology of Sex Differences. Palo Alto, Cal.: Stanford University Press.
Money, J. and Ehrhardt, A. A.
    1972 Man and Woman, Boy and Girl. Baltimore, Maryland: Johns Hopkins Press.
Parsons, T.
    1954 Essays in Sociological Theory. New York: Free Press.
Peevers, B. H. and Secord, P. F.
    1973 Developmental changes in 'Attribution of descriptive concepts to persons'. Journal of Personality and Social Psychology 27: 120–28.
Rosaldo, M. Z. and Lamphere, L.
    1974 Woman, Culture and Society. Stanford University Press.
Spence, J. and Helmreich, R.
    1978 Masculinity and Feminity. Austin, Texas: University of Texas Press.
Sullivan, H. S.
    1940 Conceptions of Modern Psychiatry. W. W. Norton.
Weitz, S.
    1977 Sex Roles. Oxford University Press.
Weizman, L. and Rizzo, D.
    1974 Biased Textbooks. Washington, D.C.: Resource Center on Sex Roles in Education.
Wolff, Kurt H.
    1974 The Sociology of Georg Simmel. The Free Press.

APPENDIX I

LIST OF AMERICAN READERS

Daystreaming (1978). The Economy Company, Oklahoma City, Oklahoma.
Keystone (1976). Houghton Mifflin Co., Boston, Mass.

Looking Around (1975). Charles E. Merrill, Columbus, Ohio.
Making Choices (1975). Charles E. Merrill, Columbus, Ohio.
Medley (1972). Houghton Mifflin, Boston, Mass.
On the Edge (1973). Ginn and Co., Lexington, Mass.
The Sun that Warms (1973). Ginn and Co., Lexington, Mass.
Tell Me How the Sun Rose (1976). Ginn and Co., Lexington, Mass.
Windows, Doorways, Bridges (1976). Scott, Foresman & Co., Glenview, Illinois.

APPENDIX II

LIST OF SWEDISH READERS

Fyran Laser (1973). Gleerup, Lund.
For Dej Ah Lasa Och Uppleva (1974). Almkuist/Wiksell, Uppsala.
Las I Egen Takt (1975). Essette Stadium, Stockholm.
Liv Och Lust (1978). Biblioteksforlaget, Stockholm.
Nu Laser Vi Vidare (1976). Almkuist/Wiksell, Uppsala.
Vad Var Det Jag Laste (1971). Gleerups, Lund.
Vi Laser (1972). Bertil Lindstro Laromedelforlagen, Essette A.B., Stockholm.

APPENDIX III

I AM A: BOY   I AM IN GRADE _____
       GIRL

LIST 3 STUDENTS IN THIS SCHOOL WHOM YOU WOULD MOST LIKE TO HAVE
HELP YOU WITH YOUR HOMEWORK, OR HELP YOU WITH A CLASS PROJECT, OR
HELP YOU WITH ANY KIND OF SCHOOLWORK. THEY MAY BE EITHER BOYS OR
GIRLS. THEY MAY BE IN YOUR CLASS OR IN ANOTHER CLASS. WRITE DOWN
ONLY THE FIRST NAMES OF THE STUDENTS YOU CHOOSE.

1. _____
2. _____
3. _____

I AM A: BOY   I AM IN GRADE _____
       GIRL

LIST 3 STUDENTS IN THIS SCHOOL WITH WHOM YOU WOULD MOST LIKE TO
SHARE A SECRET. THIS WOULD BE A SECRET THAT YOU WOULD NOT SHARE
WITH OTHER STUDENTS. THEY MAY BE EITHER BOYS OR GIRLS. THEY MAY BE
IN YOUR CLASS OR IN ANOTHER CLASS. WRITE DOWN ONLY THE FIRST NAMES
OF THE STUDENTS YOU CHOOSE.

1. _____
2. _____
3. _____

CHARLES S. DOWNING, B.Sc.

SEX DIFFERENCES IN CHILDREN'S ROAD ACCIDENTS

SUMMARY. Road accident statistics reveal that boys are more often casualties than girls. As pedestrians, this may be because boys play in the street environment more than girls, or because boys cross roads more frequently or because they do not cross roads as safely as girls. The evidence suggests that play may be the main factor associated with boys having a higher road casualty rate than girls. There is also some evidence to suggest that boys may cross roads in a slightly less safe way than girls but the evidence does not suggest that boys cross roads more often than girls.

Both parents and primary schools in the United Kingdom seem to expect and even reinforce different sex roles, such as more aggression and adventure among boys, which may account for the sex differences in road behaviour and in accident rates. However, it is difficult to determine to what extent these different parental and teacher expectancies and the different boy/girl pedestrian behaviour exhibited reflect innate differences between boys and girls or culturally determined sex stereotypes.

INTRODUCTION

Road accidents are one of the main causes of death and injury of young children, who are, unfortunately, particularly vulnerable. Road accident statistics also typically reveal that casualties are higher amongst young males than young females. In the United Kingdom (UK), children are most commonly injured on the roads as pedestrians and as pedal cyclists. Table I shows the UK casualty data for 1977 for boys and girls as pedestrians and as pedal cyclists.

TABLE I

Pedestrian and pedal cyclist casualties for boys and girls aged 0–20 years in the UK (1977)

Age (years)	Pedestrian casualties (P)		
	Boys	Girls	Boy/Girl Ratio
0–4	2,786	1,721	1.7
5–9	9,518	5,349	1.8
10–15	6,743	5,789	1.2
16–20	3,559	2,853	1.2
Total 0–20	22,606	15,612	1.4

Age (years)	Pedal Cyclist Casualties (C)		
	Boys	Girls	Boy/Girl Ratio
0–20	12,470	2,370	5.3
Total (P + C)	35,076	17,982	2.0

101

In the 0–20 year old age group, there were nearly fifty percent more male pedestrian casualties than female pedestrian casualties and there were five times as many male cycling casualties as female cycling casualties.

There are three possible reasons for there being more boy casualties than girl casualties.

(1) Boys play in the road environment both on foot and on bicycles more than girls do or in a way which is more likely to bring them into conflict with traffic.

(2) Boys spend more time as purposeful pedestrians and as purposeful cyclists than girls (i.e., they make more deliberate trips, or journeys as pedestrians and cyclists).

(3) Boys do not cope as well as girls in traffic when crossing or cycling.

Pedestrians have been much more extensively studied than cyclists and the following discussion is therefore entirely devoted to evidence from pedestrian studies.

DISCUSSION

There is considerable evidence to suggest that playing in or near the streets is one factor which may contribute to boys having more road accidents than girls.

In a study of 474 accidents involving child pedestrians aged 0–14, Grayson (1975a) found that 21 per cent of the boys were out playing when injured in a road accident as compared with only 11 per cent of the girls. These data were supported by a study of 890 accidents by Preston (1972) where 32 per cent of boys and only 16 per cent of girls were injured while playing.

Observation studies also suggest that boys play outside more than girls do. Ackermans (1972) and Guttinger (1974) observed children playing outside and found that more than 60 per cent were boys. Similar results were obtained in an unpublished study by Knighting, Colborne and Grayson at the Transport and Road Research Laboratory who observed twice as many boys playing in the roadway as girls.

A survey amongst 2,017 mothers by Sadler (1972) showed that mothers were more likely to let boys play in the street than girls (see Table II).

TABLE II
Percentage of mothers who answered 'street' when asked where
their child usually played in fine weather

Age (years)	Boys	Girls
2–4	35	31
5–8	48	40

Perhaps more surprising than the sex differences was the very high number of 2–4 year olds who were said to usually play in the street.

Playing, therefore, seems to be an important factor associated with there being more road casualties amongst boys than girls. However, the data are not sufficiently detailed to determine to what extent playing accounts for the total difference in accident levels.

There is little conclusive evidence to show that boys cross roads more than girls. One study by Howarth et al. (1974) assessed the number of unaccompanied purposeful crossings in a 24 hour period for a group of 288 boys and girls aged 5 to 10 years. For children aged 8 to 10, boys made more crossings than girls but for children aged 5 to 7 there was no difference between the sexes. However, a second study by Routledge et al. (1974) showed no significant differences between boys and girls aged 5 to 11 years.

Sadler's survey (1972) amongst 2,017 mothers of children aged 2 to 8 years revealed no differences in reported unaccompanied journeys to sweet shops or on errands for boys and girls but did indicate that girls were less likely to walk to and from school on their own (9 per cent to school, 16 per cent from school) than boys (13 per cent to school, 21 per cent from school). However, studies by De Bruijn in Holland (1976) and by Schulte and Buschges in Germany (1976) found no differences in patterns of adult accompaniment during school journeys for boys and girls, although their studies may reflect cultural differences between the UK and other European countries.

Overall, the evidence suggests that boys may make slightly more purposeful crossings than girls but that the difference if any is slight and insufficient to account for the large difference in casualty rates.

Several studies have compared the road crossing behaviour of boys and girls and have investigated the development of traffic skills in boys and girls.

Grayson's accident study (1975a) showed that boys involved in accidents were less likely to have stopped at the kerb (62 per cent had not stopped) than girls (47 per cent had not stopped). More boys were running at the time of the accident (86 per cent) than girls (75 per cent) and more boys had displayed a complete lack of attention (62 per cent) than girls (50 per cent). These data suggest that boys may have more pedestrian accidents because they cross roads in a less safe way than girls.

However, when children have been observed crossing roads unobtrusively either by observers, video or film cameras, although some sex differences have been found, the evidence does not conclusively demonstrate that boys cross roads in a less safe way than girls.

Observation studies by Routledge et al. (1976), Finlayson (1972), Limbourg (1976) and Grayson (1975b) all found some evidence to indicate that girls are relatively more likely than boys to stop at the kerb before crossing and also that girls tend to make more head movements at the kerb than boys do, but these differences were not consistent from one observation site to another or for different age groups. Limbourg (1976) concluded that there

were no signficant differences in road crossing behaviour between boys and
girls.

In the Routledge et al. (1976) study, boys (aged 0 to 15) were observed to
cross in much smaller gaps in the traffic than girls (aged 0 to 15). Twenty five
per cent of boys crossed in a 3 second gap and 48 per cent in a 4 second gap.
This compared with 16 per cent of girls crossing in a 3 second gap and 32 per
cent in a 4 second gap. Nobody crossed in a gap of less than 3 seconds.

Some researchers have attempted to grade crossing behaviour from good
to bad or from safe to unsafe. Sandels (1975) found that girls exhibited better
crossing behaviour than boys and Routledge et al. (1976) found that girls
were more likely to use a 'safe' crossing strategy than boys.

Boys may therefore be slightly less cautious or safe than girls when crossing
the road but this does not seem to be associated with any underlying lesser ability
in boys to cross the road safely, a lesser knowledge of road safety (e.g., Sandels
(1975), Fisk and Cliffe (1975)) or a slower development of relevant perceptual
abilities in boys (Sandels (1975), Salvatore (1973)). The slightly less safe crossing
behaviour observed amongst boys may therefore be based on boys failing to
put into practice the behavioural rules they have learnt for crossing roads safely
as consistently as girls.

Overall, the evidence from pedestrian studies suggests that playing in or
near the street may be the main factor contributing to there being more road
casualties amongst boys than girls. There is also some evidence to indicate that
boys crossing roads in a less safe way than girls may be a factor, but there is
little evidence to suggest that boys cross roads more frequently than girls.

It is difficult to assess to what extent the differences in types of road behaviour exhibited by boys and girls reflect culturally determined sex stereotypes
or innate sex differences.

As far as road safety education is concerned there is no evidence to suggest
that boys receive different road safety instruction either in the home (Sadler
(1972)) or at Primary schools. In fact, studies by Fisk and Cliffe (1975) and
Sandels (1975) showed that boys and girls performed equally well in road crossing tests both before and after road safety instruction and that education, as
far as improving road safety knowledge is concerned, is not biased either in
favour of boys or in favour of girls.

However, there does seem to be a difference in general expectations about
boys' and girls' behaviour amongst both parents and teachers and consequently
in the activities that boys and girls are encouraged to do. In the Sadler (1972)
study, mothers of 2 to 4 year old boys were more likely to say that their child
was able to cross the road than mothers of 2 to 4 year old girls, (see Table III).

Similarly mothers were more likely to let boys play in the street (see Table II)
and to let boys go to school on their own than girls.

Avery (1974) suggested that "boys are more vulnerable to pedestrian accidents
because Australian males are encouraged to exhibit many of the aggressive
characteristics observed in accident repeating children". He put forward the

TABLE III
Percentage of children said to be able to cross the road outside their own home

Sex	Age (years)		
	2	3	4
Boys	33	50	69
Girls	19	45	58

hypothesis that "stereotyped Australian male characteristics and vulnerability to traffic accidents are in some way related".

A similar view was expressed by Klein (1976) who suggested that boys are encouraged to be competitive, aggressive and take risks in order that they might survive and succeed in a competitive and aggressive adult world.

Teachers in Primary schools also seem to expect and encourage boys and girls to behave in different ways (e.g., Department of Education and Science (1975), Lobban (1975), Weiner (1978)). Weiner (1978) wrote concerning Primary Schools that "Girls are universally rewarded for neatness, conformity and quietness, whilst boys are expected to be noisy, enthusiastic and adventurous", differences which seem likely to result in more dangerous roadside play and in less safe crossing behaviour on the part of boys.

These types of attitude and discriminatory practice on the part of parents and teachers could possibly account for the different road behaviour and higher accident rate amongst boys.

However, the extent to which these sex discriminatory attitudes and actions on the part of parents and schools and the extent to which the different road behaviours exhibited by boys and girls reflect culturally determined sex stereotypes or possible innate differences between the sexes, such as a greater exploratory drive and greater innate aggression amongst boys, would seem to be an insoluble problem.

CONCLUSION

In the United Kingdom, there are about twice as many pedestrian and cycling casualties amongst boys as there are amongst girls.

As far as pedestrians are concerned, one factor that seems to be associated with this accident difference is the fact that boys play more than girls in the street environment. There is also some evidence to suggest that boys may cross roads in a slightly less safe way than girls but the evidence does not show that boys cross roads more often than girls.

It is difficult to assess to what extent the different road behaviour exhibited by boys and girls reflects innate differences between boys and girls or culturally determined sex stereotypes. Certainly, parents and teachers seem to expect and encourage different behaviours amongst boys and girls, but these in turn may reflect innate differences between boys and girls or culturally determined sex stereotypes or both.

Department of Transport, England

ACKNOWLEDGEMENT

The work described in this paper forms part of the programme of the Transport and Road Research Laboratory and the paper is published by permission of the Director.

Any views expressed in this paper are not necessarily those of the Department of the Environment or of the Department of Transport. Extracts from the text may be reproduced, except for commercial purposes, provided the source is acknowledged.

REFERENCES

Ackermans, E.
  1972 De woonomgeving als speelgelegenheid. Groningen, The Netherlands: Wolters-Noordhof.
Avery, G. C.
  1974 The capacity of young children to cope with the traffic system: a review. Traffic Accident Research Unit, Department of Motor Transport, New South Wales.
Bruijn, T. G. de
  1976 Schoolroutes van kinderen. Verkeersbureau Amsterdam.
Department of Education and Science
  1975 Curricular differences for boys and girls. Educational Survey 21. London: HMSO.
Finlayson, H. M.
  1972 Children's road behaviour and personality. Department of Psychology. The University of Southampton.
Grayson, G. B.
  1975a The Hampshire child pedestrian accident study. Department of the Environment. Transport and Road Research Laboratory. Laboratory report 688.
Grayson, G. B.
  1975b Observations of pedestrian behaviour at four sites. Department of the Environment. Transport and Road Research Laboratory. Laboratory report 670.
Guttinger, V. A.
  1974 De gebruikswaarde van de woonomgeving. N.I.P.G.–T.N.O. Leiden, The Netherlands.
Howarth, C. I., Routledge, D. A., and Repetto-Wright, R.
  1974 An analysis of road accidents involving child pedestrians. Ergonomics 17: 319–330.
Klein, D.
  1976 Who is to blame for childhood injuries. Safety Education 137: 3–5.
Limbourg, M.
  1976 Das Verhalten von 4–9 jährigen Kindern bei der Strassenüberquerung. Zeitschrift für experimentelle und angewandte Psychologie 23: 666–77.
Lobban G.
  1975 Sexism in primary school. Women Speaking, 4 July.

Molen, H. H. van der
  1976 Observational studies of children's road crossing behaviour: a review of the literature. Traffic Research Centre. Rijksuniversiteit Groningen, The Netherlands.
Preston, B.
  1972 Statistical Analysis of child pedestrian accidents in Manchester and Salford. Accid. Anal. and Prev. 4: 323–332.
Routledge, D. A., Repetto-Wright, R., and Howarth, C. I.
  1974 A comparison of interviews and observation to obtain measures of children's exposure to risk as pedestrians, Ergonomics 17: 623–638.
Routledge, D. A., Repetto-Wright, R., and Howarth, C. I.
  1976 The development of road crossing skill by child pedestrians. Paper presented to the International Conference on Pedestrian Safety, Haifa, Israel, 1976.
Sadler, J.
  1972 Children and road safety: A survey amongst mothers. Office of population censuses and surveys, London: HMSO.
Salvatore, S.
  1973 The ability of elementary and secondary school children to sense oncoming car velocity. Highway Research Record 436: 19–28.
Sandels, S.
  1975 Children in Traffic. London: Paul Elek.
Schulte, W., and Buschges, G.
  1976 Strassenverkehrsbeteiligung von Kindern and Jugendlichen. Arbeitsgruppe Verkehrssicherheitsforschung an der Fakultät für soziologie der Universität Bielefeld.
Weiner, G.
  1978 Education and the Sex Discrimination Act. Educational Research 20: 163–173.

SOPHIA M. R. LEUNG, M.S.W. and BETTY KLEIMAN, M.D.

CULTURAL DIFFERENCES IN CHILDREN'S SEX ROLE STEREOTYPES

INTRODUCTION

Considerable attention has been focussed on the exploration of human sex role development. Knowledge of sex role stereotypes begins very early. Kubu (1978) and his colleagues have indicated that two to three year old children possess substantial knowledge of those sex role stereotypes predominant in the adult culture. Mussen (1969) demonstrated that behaviours of sex role sterotypes are pronounced in four to five year old children. Money and Ehrhardt (1972) asserted that a child's sex identity is psychologically irreversible after the age of three years. Knowledge of sex role and sex identity are integrated very early in personality development.

When children first develop sex role stereotypes is known, but how this process is formulated is unclear. Brush and Goldberg (1977) indicated in their study that pre-school children do not show a consistent pattern of sex role behaviour. Researchers have found that cranial hair and clothes are the most important discriminating cues for children younger than four years, supported by Levin (1972), and Thompson (1975). Young children's discriminating ability for sex differences may come some time after learning the sex gender labels and cues as Thompson and Bentler (1973) suggested. One theory of sex role development is proposed by Kohlberg (1966). He suggested a cognitive development theory as the basis of sex role development, and this is supported by Marcus and Overton (1978). So sex role stereotypes may be perceived as a complex physical, psychosocial developmental process in a young child. The major determining factors are unclear.

Since society and culture play an important role in influencing a child's perception of sexual identity, we wondered how children from different cultural backgrounds develop ideas of masculine and feminine roles. Were there definite cultural factors affecting the children's sex role stereotypes, and how?

Downing (1975) noted the cultural differences in children's concept of learning in kindergarten groups of Canadian Indian and non-Indian children by measuring their differences in literacy activities and technical knowledge of speech and writing. Leung (1977) studied grade seven students in the People's Republic of China. The personal aspiration and career selection of the Chinese boys and girls were surprisingly similar without sex role discrimination. From cross-cultural studies we recognize that cultural differences influence the concept of sex roles. The purpose of this study is to examine the relationship between cultural differences and the development of sex role stereotypes. Similarities and differences in the young children's concept of sex roles in different cultural contexts will be determined. The aim of our study is to obtain further indications of the effects

I. Gross, J. Downing, and A. d'Heurle (eds.), Sex Role Attitudes and Cultural Change, 109–120.
Copyright © 1982 by D. Reidel Publishing Company.

of different cultural backgrounds on children's sex role development. It investigates a child's ability to recognize certain psychological characteristics, attributes or behaviours as typically masculine and feminine within a culturally determined sample.

METHOD

Subjects

The children studied were from three different cultural backgrounds: Chinese, Jewish and Anglo-Saxon Canadians in Vancouver. All children were 4 1/2 to 5 1/2 years old or 54 to 66 months.

Chinese Group

Children in this study are usually the offspring of the first generation in Canada. The parents or the children were born in China or Asia. The family retains mainly Chinese tradition and values. They speak Chinese dialects at home, using limited English. We selected these children from Chinese Day care programmes which presented Western styled pre-school activities by a mixed Chinese and Canadian staff. A Chinese staff helped to interpret the testing material when the child had limited English skills.

Jewish Group

Children were defined as culturally Jewish if the parents are identified culturally and religiously as Jewish. These children were also enrolled in a Jewish day-care programme organized by Vancouver Jewish Community Centre.

Canadian Group

Children selected for our Canadian sample were white Anglo-Saxons and English-speaking, as their first language at home. These children also attend local Day-Care Programmes.

Selection of Day-Care Programmes

Day-Care Programmes were selected on the basis of their cultural orientation, location and availability in our community. The testing arrangements were independently made by the authors, the parents and the Day-Care teachers. The teachers also completed a questionnaire to provide demographic information.

PROCEDURES

Sex Stereotype Measure (SSM)

The 4 1/2 to 5 1/2 year old children were administered the SSM II procedure individually. The Sex Stereotype Measure is a picture-story test developed by Williams, Bennett and Best (1975) to assess children's knowledge of adult-defined sex role stereotypes. They revised the original material to produce the SSM II. It is a tested procedure employing 32 story-pictures designed to represent characteristic traits which adults define as the stereotypes of masculine and feminine. These stereotypes have little relationship to physiological differences between men and women.

The SSM II procedure has been used in the United States, England, Ireland, with 5, 8 and 11 year olds, reportedly by Williams et al. (1977). Additional tests have been done in the Netherlands, France and Japan. Studies are presently under way in Australia, Bolivia, Brazil, Canada, Chile, West Germany, Greece, South Nigeria, India, Israel, Italy, New Zealand, Norway, Pakistan, Peru, Scotland, South Africa, Sweden, Taiwan and Venezuela.

Testing Procedure

The testing material consists of:

1. 32 pairs of human silhouettes (16 AS AND 16 BS) one male and one female, presented in a variety of postures. The A and B pictures are presented alternately to the children.

2. There are 32 stories to accompany each pair of the male-female pictures. The 16 Group A were randomized with the 16 Group B pictures and the orders of the pictures were arranged randomly as AB, BA, so that no individual subject would have the same sequence.

3. Following a brief initial conversation designed to put the subject at ease, the examiner gave the following instructions for the SSM II: "What I have here are some pictures I would like to show you and some stories that go with each one. I want you to help me by pointing to the person in each picture that the story is about. Here — I will show you what I mean." Then the examiner would display the first picture and read the first story.

4. The examiner will record the subject's responses on an answer sheet (see Appendix). The subject selected the figure following each story.

Following the completion of the test, the examiner said to the subject, "Thank you for playing the games with me and I would appreciate it if you would not talk to the other children about the game we have played here so that the game will be new to them too."

Recording of Score

The subject's response to SSM II was scored by the total number of stereotype scores. A female stereotype score was counted by one point for each of the 16 female items selected by the subject's choice of a female figure. A male stereotype score was obtained on the same basis by counting one point for selecting a male figure in response to each of the 16 male items. Each of these stereotype subscores had a range of 0–16 points. High scores indicate a high degree of stereotype knowledge, low scores indicating no knowledge of or a reversal of conventional stereotypes. The combination of the male and female stereotype subscores make up the total stereotype score, with a range of 0–32 points and a chance midpoint of 16.

RESULTS

For our study we tested 80 pre-school children from predominantly middle-class families. The total group consisted of 40 male and 40 female children with the ages of 4 1/2 to 5 1/2 years.

The children can be presented as the following cultural groups (see Table I):

1.   10 male Chinese children
      10 female
2.   10 male Jewish children
      10 female
3.   10 male white Anglo-Saxon Canadian children
      10 female
4.   10 male white Anglo-Saxon Canadian Single-Parent children
      10 female white Anglo-Saxon Canadian Single-Parent children

TABLE I

Summary of sample categories used for data analysis

80 Preschool Children							
20 Jewish		20 Chinese		20 Canadian Single Parent		20 Canadian 2 Parent	
10 male	10 female	10 male	10 female	10 male	10 female	10 male	10 female

DATA ANALYSIS:
CROSS CULTURAL COMPARISON OF THE MEAN SCORE

Each cultural group presented in Table II has the basic variance of (1) cultural group of subject (2) subject's different selection of male and female stereotype score and the total score.

The findings of Table II presenting the 80 children's six stereotypes of the three cultural groups can be summarized as follows:

(1) The 80 children evidently showed awareness and knowledge of sex stereotypes at the age of 4½ to 5½ years.

(2) There are some differences of sex stereotypes among the boys and girls.

TABLE II

Cross cultural comparison: Means of male (M), female (F), and total (T) sex role stereotype (SSM II) scores among 5 year old children

	N	M	F	T
Chinese				
Boys	10	10.0	8.8	18.8
Girls	10	9.4	7.7	17.1
Total	20	9.7	8.3	17.9
Jewish				
Boys	10	9.5	7.4	16.9
Girls	10	8.6	9.4	18.0
Total	20	9.1	8.4	17.5
Canadian (Two parents)				
Boys	10	10.2	9.3	19.5
Girls	10	8.5	8.7	17.2
Total	20	9.4	9.0	18.4
Canadian (Single parent)				
Boys	10	8.8	8.8	17.6
Girls	10	9.3	9.3	18.6
Total	20	9.1	9.1	18.1
Total Children				
Boys	40	9.6	8.6	18.2
Girls	40	9.0	8.8	17.7
Total	80	9.3	8.7	18.0

(3) Male stereotypes appeared more developed than female stereotypes in all the children of Chinese, Jewish and Canadian background.

(4) Both the Chinese and Jewish children appeared to be less aware of the female stereotype in comparison with the Canadian groups. Perhaps the female role was diffused and unclear to the Chinese and Jewish subjects.

(5) The Canadian children (with two parents) had slightly higher total score of sex stereotypes. Perhaps they have acquired more awareness and knowledge of sex stereotypes than the other groups.

(6) The Chinese children showed a more developed male stereotype. The Jewish boys had less knowledge of female stereotype.

(7) There was similar responses of sex stereotypes between the Canadian children with 2 parents and the Canadian children with single parents. The mean scores of Canadian children (2 parents) were Male–Female 9.4 : 9.0, with total mean of 18.4. And the mean scores of Canadian children (single parent) were Male–Female 9.1 : 9.1, with total mean of 18.1.

(8) The total mean scores: Chinese 17.9, Jewish 17.5, Canadian (2 parents) 18.4, and Canadian (single parent) 18.4. So the Chinese and Jewish children are less sex stereotyped than the Canadian children (by Canadian standards).

CHILDREN'S RESPONSES TO SEX STEREOTYPE BY CROSS CULTURAL COMPARISON

From Table III we will examine the data which was presented as percent of the subject's stereotyped responses to each of the 32 SSM II items (e.g., emotional, aggressive, strong, etc.). In Table III all stereotypes of 67% or higher and 33% or lower were italicized.

TABLE III

Percent of 5 year old children expressed stereotyped responses to each SSM II item by cross cultural comparison

Item Stereotype Traits No. (Adult Definition)	Chinese (N-20)	Jewish (N-20)	Canadian (N-20)	Canadian S.P.[a] (N-20)	Total (N-80)
1. emotional	50	60	60	45	54
2. aggressive, assertive	50	70	60	45	56
3. adventurous	40	35	75	60	53
4. appreciative	40	60	70	35	51
5. weak	55	70	75	65	66
6. independent	60	80	40	60	60
7. disorderly	65	55	40	50	53
8. talkative	55	40	50	50	49
9. fickle, rattle-brained	55	45	30	55	46
10. ambitious, enterprising	25	50	60	75	53
11. jolly	70	60	50	50	58
12. gentle	55	75	40	60	58
13. frivolous	45	40	65	70	55
14. cruel	70	70	65	70	69
15. steady, stable	80	50	45	50	38
16. fussy, nagging	45	30	40	70	46
17. meek, mild	45	55	75	60	59
18. boastful	55	50	60	70	59
19. coarse	65	55	60	50	58
20. whiny, complaining	70	40	50	55	54
21. flirtatious, charming	35	55	40	50	45
22. severe, stern	60	60	65	30	54
23. loud	65	70	65	65	66
24. excitable, high strung	55	65	65	60	61
25. affectionate	55	85	75	40	64
26. dominant, autocratic	50	55	75	55	59
27. self-confident, confident	75	45	55	60	59
28. sentimental, soft hearted	75	45	55	60	59
29. dependent, submissive	55	55	50	35	49
30. logical, rational	65	65	55	35	55
31. strong, robust	65	85	85	80	79
32. sophisticated, affected	70	70	60	45	61

[a] Canadian children with a single parent.
All stereotypes of 66% or higher and 33% or lower are in italics.

The results of this data can be analysed as in Table IV:

TABLE IV
Cross cultural comparison of 80 five year old children's responses to sex stereotype

Subject	Chinese	Jewish	Canadian (2 P.)	Canadian (S.P.)
Female stereotype	Complaining Sophisticated*	Weak Gentle Affectionate* Sophisticated*	Appreciative Weak Affectionate* Meek	Frivolous Fussy
Male Stereotype	Jolly Cruel Confident	Aggressive Independent Loud Strong*	Adventurous Dominant Strong*	Ambitious Cruel Boastful Strong*
Role Reversals	Female- Ambitious	Male- Fussy		Female- Severe

* Same stereotype shared by the above groups.

The data in Table IV shows the stereotypes of 67% or higher and 33% or lower as the role reversal.

Chinese subjects: Found that women are "complaining, sentimental and sophisticated" while men are "jolly, cruel and confident". We noted that Chinese subjects indicated a role reversal where they think women are more ambitious than men.

Jewish subjects: They found that the women are "weak, gentle, affectionate and sophisticated" while men are "aggressive, independent, loud and strong" with one role reversal in believing male to be fussier than the female. The total number of stereotypes was 8 (4 male and 4 female).

Canadian subjects with 2 parents: They felt that women are "appreciative, meek and affectionate" while men are "adventurous, dominant and strong".

Canadian subjects with single parent: They thought that women were "frivolous and fussy" while men were "ambitious, cruel, boastful and strong". There was one role reversal where females were found to be more severe than men. Interesting to note that the children in this group were generally living with their single mother at home.

In summary, the Chinese strongly identified 6 (3 female, 3 male) out of 32 stereotypes, having only 1 role reversal as 3% of the total stereotypes. The Jewish highly recognized 8 (4 male and 4 female) stereotypes, without role reversal. The Canadians with 2 parents, identified 6 (3 female, 3 male) of the stereotypes. And the Canadians with single parent, identified 6 (2 female, 4 male) of the total stereotypes with 3% as role reversal. All other stereotypes fell into a chance level of responses (34%–66%).

PERCENT OF MALE (M), FEMALE (F), AND TOTAL (T) FIVE YEAR OLD CHILDREN'S STEREOTYPED RESPONSES

From Table V (16 female items of SSM II) and Table VI (16 male items), we will analyze in Table VII the 80 subjects' sex stereotypes in terms of the boys' and girls' identification of the male and female items of the SSM II procedure.

It is interesting to note that the boys and girls closely identified women as "talkative, fickle and dependent", men as "independent, cruel, steady, loud" with the similar scores on the female items and male items in Tables V and VI.

TABLE V

Percent of male (M), female (F), and total (T) children's expressed stereotyped responses to 32 SSM II items

Item No.	Stereotype Traits (Adult Definition)	M (N–40)	F (N–40)	T (N–80)
Female Items		%	%	%
1.	emotional	48	58	53
4.	appreciative	55	48	51
5.	weak	70	63	66
8.	talkative	45	48	46
9.	fickle, rattle-brained	45	43	44
12.	gentle	55	60	58
13.	frivolous	58	50	54
16.	fussy	50	43	46
17.	meek, mild	58	63	60
20.	whiny, complaining	53	60	56
21.	flirtatious, charming	33	58	45
24.	excitable	65	60	63
25.	affectionate	70	55	63
28.	sentimental	63	55	59
29.	dependent, submissive	48	48	48
32.	sophisticated, affected	50	75	63

TABLE VI

Percent of male (M), female (F), and total (T) children expressed stereotyped responses to each SSM II item

Item No.	Stereotype Traits (Adult Definition)	M (N−40)	F (N−40)	T (N−80)
Male Items		%	%	%
2.	aggressive, assertive	53	60	56
3.	adventurous	65	40	53
6.	independent	65	63	64
7.	disorderly	55	50	53
10.	ambitious, enterprising	68	60	64
11.	jolly	55	60	58
14.	cruel	70	70	70
15.	steady, stable	58	55	56
18.	boastful	48	73	60
19.	coarse	48	68	58
22.	severe, stern	58	50	54
23.	loud	65	68	66
26.	dominant, autocratic	70	48	59
27.	self-confident, confident	70	53	61
30.	logical	63	45	54
31.	strong, robust	85	73	79

TABLE VII

	Five year old boys (N−40)	Five year old girls (N−40)	Five year old boys & girls (N−80)
Female Items	weak affectionate	sophisticated	weak
Male Items	ambitious cruel dominant self-confident strong	cruel boastful coarse loud strong	cruel loud strong
Role Reversals	male-flirtatious		

We have selected stereotypes of 67% or higher, 33% or lower as role reversals to be illustrated above. The girls strong recognized women as "sophisticated" and men as "cruel, boastful, coarse, loud and strong". The boys firmly believed that women were "weak, affectionate" and men were "ambitious, cruel, dominant, self-confident and strong" plus one role reversal finding men more "flirtatious" than women. When we examined the joint beliefs of both the boys and girls, they recognized that women are "weak" and men are "cruel, loud and strong". They shared one stereotype by all identifying men as "strong".

DISCUSSION

Our study has demonstrated that human sex stereotyping develops rather early in life. Our sample of 80 pre-school children showed clear awareness and knowledge of sex stereotypes at ages of 4½ to 5½ years. They had established views of those masculine and feminine roles which predominate in our adult society. This finding is in agreement with the suggestion of Best, Williams, and Cloud et al. (1977). However the children were not in complete agreement regarding the characteristics of sex role stereotypes. The differences appear to be related to cultural background.

For instance, it appears that the Chinese and Jewish subjects seemed to be less aware of the female stereotype than the Caucasian Canadian children. We may speculate that the latter's families of the Chinese and Jewish children produced a more diffused image. The Chinese children believed that women are "complaining, sophisticated" and more "ambitious" than men. These terms are, in Canadian society, applied to men. The Jewish children indicated that the women are "weak, gentle, affectionate and sophisticated" while men are thought to be more fussy than women. Again this is an interesting role reversal from traditional sex roles.

Those Caucasian Canadian children with two parents predominantly recognized that women are "appreciative, meek, affectionate" while those children with only a mother felt that women are "frivolous, fussy" and more "severe" than men. Lack of a father-figure in these families and the assumption by the mother of both the female and male roles may account for this. It is understandable that these children perceived their mothers as being fussy and severe since they have to undertake both the disciplinary and breadwinning roles. On the other hand there were a number of similar responses of sex stereotypes given by both groups of children. It would be of interest to make further comparative study of these two different social groups.

When we compare the sex stereotyping by the 40 boys with the 40 girls, we found that the boys more frequently identified the women as "meek and affectionate" and men as "ambitious, cruel, dominant, self-confident and strong". Men were also described as being more "flirtatious" than women. The 40 girls believed that women are "sophisticated" while men "cruel, boastful, coarse, loud and strong". Certainly the boys and girls differed markedly in their view of masculine and feminine characteristics.

It is obvious that some of the children's descriptions represented the traditionally rigid judgement and sex discriminatory viewpoint. However, the children acquired these unhealthy stereotypes in early childhood because of the role modeling by the adults they encountered in their daily life. Their parents, relatives, friends, teachers and workers at the day-care centres are all part of the powerful influential agents which affect these young and impressionable children. Adults must be alert and be aware of the differences and disparity between healthy sex roles and discriminatory ones. Further study should also be focused upon cross cultural differences in children's awareness of sex discrimination.

So far we have only examined children from 4½ to 5½ years of age. It may prove valuable to extend this study to include 8 and 11 year olds, and from different cultural groups.

Finally, we think that basic information on sex role development and its determinants may be key elements for gaining understanding and a pathway to acquire a healthy attitude towards masculine and feminine roles.

Vancouver General Hospital

ACKNOWLEDGEMENT

We thank Pam Tobe, Phyllis Redekop, Alison Miller and Elaine Ho for their assistance in this study.

REFERENCES

Best, D. L., Williams, J. E., Cloud, J. M., Davis, S. W., Robertson, L. S., Edwards, J. R., Giles, H., and Fowles, J.
  1977 Development of sex-trait stereotypes among young children in the United States, England, and Ireland. Child Development 48: 1375–1384.
Brush, L. R. and Goldberg, W. A.
  1977 The intercorrelation of measures of sex-role identity. J. Child Psychol., Psychiat. 19: 43–48.
Downing, J., Ollila, L., and Oliver, P.
  1975 Cultural differences in children's concepts of reading and writing. Br. J. Educ. Psychol. 45: 312–316.
Kohlberg, L. A.
  1966 A cognitive-developmental analysis of children's sex-role concepts and attitudes. in E. Maccoby (ed.), The Development of Sex Differences. Stanford: Stanford University Press.
Kubu, D., Nash, S. C., and Brucken, L.
  1978 Sex role concepts of two and three year olds. Child Development 49: 445–451.
Leung, S. M. R.
  1977 Sex roles of children in the People's Republic of China. Proceedings of the World Congress of Mental Health, Vancouver, Canada.
Levin, S. M., Balistrieri, J., and Schukit, M.
  1972 The development of sexual discrimination in children. J. of Child Psychol, and Psychiat. 13: 47–53.
Marcus, D. E. and Overton, W. F.
  1978 The development of cognitive gender consistency and sex role preferences. Child Development 49: 434–444.
Money, J. and Ehrhardt, A. A.
  1972 Man and Woman, Boy and Girl. Baltimore: John Hopkins University Press.

Mussen, P. H.
  1969 Early sex-role development in D. A. Goslin (ed.), Handbook of Socialization
        Theory and Research: Chicago: Rand-McNally.
Thompson, S. K.
  1975 Gender labels and early sex role development. Child Development 46: 339–347.
Thompson, S. K. and Bentler, P. M.
  1973 A developmental study of gender constancy and parent preference. Archives of
        Sexual Behaviour 2: 379–385.
Williams, J. E. and Bennett, S. M.
  1975 The definition of sex stereotypes via the adjective check list. Sex Roles 1: 327–
        337.

SOLLY B. DREMAN, Ph.D.

SEX ROLE STEREOTYPING AND MENTAL HEALTH
STANDARDS IN ISRAEL: A CROSS-CULTURAL COMPARISON

Sex role stereotyping in mental health standards in Israel in a sample of 60 non-clients, 60 clients, 60 psychotherapists were investigated. Recent studies of sex role stereotypes in America have shown that males still maintain traditional stereotypes and perceive the healthy adult female as more stereotypically feminine than either the healthy male or adult. Women, however, have changed their traditional perceptions toward female mental health and now rate the healthy adult female as similar to the healthy adult male and the healthy adult. In contrast to the recent American findings, female therepists in the Israeli study viewed the healthy female as significantly more stereotypically feminine than the healthy male. Male therapists were more equalitarian in their ratings and surprisingly rated the healthy male as significantly more feminine than did female therapists. These findings are discussed in terms of cross-cultural differences. Congruency of client-therapist sex-linked mental health standards is also examined and the implications for the therapeutic process discussed. Some of the faults in the research conducted on sex stereotypes are noted.

Sex stereotyping has become of increasing concern to the helping professions because stereotyping may be psychologically damaging and hinder development. This may be particularly acute for women because sex role stereotyping has been shown to depress their vocational aspirations (Epstein, 1970), cause psychic conflict with regard to achievement (Horner, 1968), precipitate mental illness (Chesler, 1972), and contribute to the devaluation of their own sex (Rosenkrantz, Vogel, Bee, Broverman, and Broverman, 1968). Earlier studies of mental health standards have shown that mental health clinicians maintain a double standard of mental health for the sexes. Broverman, Broverman, Clarkson, Rosenkrantz, and Vogel (1970), for example, asked psychiatrists, psychologists, and social workers to describe a "healthy, mature, socially competent adult man," "a healthy, mature, socially competent adult woman," and "a healthy, mature, socially competent adult" (sex not specified) using the Rosenkrantz et al. (1968) Sex Stereotype Questionnaire. They found that both female and male clinicians had different concepts of health for men vs. women. The concept for a healthy man was parallel to the concept of a healthy adult (sex not specified), but the healthy woman was described as differing from males and adults in general and as more submissive, more easily influenced, less independent, more emotional and less objective. It is interesting to note that both female and male clinicians adopted identical sex biases in the above study.

The growing influence of the women's liberation movement has led to public reassessment of sex roles and spurred recent research in this area. Maslin and Davis (1975), for example, who used the Rosenkrantz et al. (1968) Stereotype

I. Gross, J. Downing, and A. d'Heurle (eds.), Sex Role Attitudes and Cultural Change, 121–129.
Copyright © 1982 by D. Reidel Publishing Company.

Questionnaire on a group of counselors-in-training, found that female counselors, in contrast to the earlier Broverman et al. (1970) study, perceived healthy females as similar to healthy males and adults in general. Similarly, Kravetz (1970) studied the sex role concepts of 150 university women with the Rosenkrantz et al. questionnaire and found that their perceptions of female mental health had changed and were significantly more "masculine" than previously identified. A recent study by Deutsch and Gilbert (1976) suggests that in fact masculine behavior may be compatible with mental health in American women. Thus the college women who described themselves as masculine on the Bem Sex Role Inventory were better adjusted relative to other women.

While the above evidence suggests some change in females' perceptions of mental health, this is less apparent for males. Male counselors in the Maslin and Davis (1975) study, for example, rated healthy males and adults in general as similar, but still maintained the traditional stereotypically feminine standard for female mental health. Similarly, a task force set up in 1974 by the Board of Professional Affairs of the American Psychological Association to examine sex bias and sex role stereotypes as they affect women as students, practitioners and consumers of psychotherapy found that male therapists actively employ sexist notions in therapy by encouraging females to be less career oriented and assertive and to find self-actualization in their roles as mother and wife. Male therapists who try to keep their female clients in "their place," however, may be doing them an injustice if such behavior results in poorer adjustment, as Deutsch and Gilbert's (1976) recent study suggests.

The present research intends to replicate and extend the earlier work of Maslin and Davis (1975) on therapists' sex-stereotypes toward mental health. Thus in addition to a therapist population, the present study also will investigate a client population and a control group of nonclients with regard to their sex-stereotypes of mental health. In addition, we are cross-culturally extending the Maslin and Davis research to an Israeli population. The research is a 3 X 2 X 3 factorial design: rater (nonclients, clients, therapists) X rater sex (male, female) X ratee sex (healthy adult, healthy male, healthy female). The inclusion of a client population will permit us to examine congruency of client vs. therapist stereotypes of mental health in addition to rater sex differences in mental health stereotypes.

METHOD

Subjects

Participants were 60 psychotherapists, 60 clients of psychotherapy, and 60 nonclients who never had been in therapy. Psychotherapists were canvassed from various university counseling services as well as from registers of social workers, psychologists, and psychiatrists in Israel. Questionnaires were administered individually to them. Questionnaires were accepted on a quota basis and sampling stopped when a sample of 30 male and 30 female therapists was attained. The final sample consisted of 7 psychiatrists, 39 psychologists and 12 social workers (2 Ss did not indicate professional affiliation). In a 3 X 2 X 3 analysis of variance: profession X rater sex X ratee sex, no main or interaction effects were found for profession on sex stereotype scores. Because the Maslin and Davis (1975) study used counselors-in-training while the present study utilized both trainees and senior therapists, "therapist status" was treated as an independent variable and therapists were dichotomized as either "seniors" (N = 36), those who had completed an internship in psychotherapy in an accredited training institute and had at least 2 years' post internship experience, or "juniors" (N = 24), those who were still undergoing training in an accredited institution. A 2 X 2 X 3 analysis of variance: therapist status X rater sex X ratee sex, showed no main or interaction effects for therapist status on sex stereotype scores.

Clients consisted of students who had approached an Israeli university student counseling service for counseling. All new prospective clients were tested before the initial intake session, and sampling continued until the quota of 30 male and 30 female clients was reached. Nonclients included the first 30 male and 30 female students of an Israeli university who were approached and had indicated that they had never received psychotherapy or psychological counseling. Admittedly this sample is not random; however, all Ss approached agreed to answer the questionnaire, which ruled out such factors as self-selection as possible intervening variables. The mean age was nonclients 22.9; clients 24.2; therapists 35.3.

Instrument

A shortened version of the Stereotype Questionnaire (Rosenkrantz et al., 1968) was used, which included 38 items that previously had been established as sex stereotypic among both male and female college students and also judged suitable for use with mental health clinicians (Broverman et al., 1970). Items are presented as bipolar traits, such as:

> Not at all self-confident . . . . Very self-confident
> Very tactful . . . . Very blunt

Each item is evaluated by the respondent on a scale from 1 to 7; certain items appear with poles reversed to reduce response set. Items were scored so that the lower end of the pole (score of 1) indicated extreme stereotypically feminine behavior, while the higher end (score of 7) indicated extreme stereotypically masculine behavior. Although Broverman et al. (1970) scored the 38 stereotypic items only in terms of directionality from the midpoint toward either pole, we recorded a numerical score for each item as marked on the scale. Thus group mean scores in this study are the average total scores within each group. This permitted us to compare more readily our results with Maslin and Davis'

(1975) study, which adopted identical scoring procedures. It should be noted
that a high total score is indicative of more stereotypically masculine behavior.

Procedure

Ss within each major population were assigned randomly by sex to one of three
sets of instruction (healthy adult, healthy male, healthy female). The study was
thus a complete 3 × 2 × 3 factorial design: rater (nonclients, clients, therapists)
× rater sex × ratee sex (healthy adult, healthy male, healthy female) with 10
Ss in each of the 18 cells of the design. Ss received the following instructions:

We would like to know something about what people expect other people to be like. Imagine
that you are going to meet someone for the first time and the only thing you know in
advance is that the person is a *healthy, mature, socially competent adult* (or *healthy, mature,
socially competent adult male*, or *healthy, mature, socially competent adult female* depending on which instruction condition the subject was assigned). What sort of things would
you expect? For example, what would you expect about the person's liking or disliking of
the color red? Put a circle on the scale according to what you think the person is like. For
example:

Strong dislike for   Strong liking for
the color red 1 . . . . . . 2 . . . . . . 3 . . . . . .   the color red
          4 . . . . . . 5 . . . . . . 6 7

On the following pages are a number of scales like the one above. Please place a circle at
the point you expect a *healthy, mature, socially competent adult* (or *healthy, mature,
socially competent male* or *healthy, mature, socially competent female*) to be like. You
may put your choice anywhere on the scale, not just at the numbers.

PLEASE BE SURE TO MARK EVERY ITEM.

Ss were assured of anonymity and were unaware tnat they had received different instructions or that sex stereotyping was being investigated. Within the
limits of the 38 stereotypic items, responses to the *adult* (sex unspecified)
instructions can be considered indicative of this sample's standard of mental
health for adults, irrespective of sex. Responses to *adult male* instructions
provide a measure of their standard for male mental health, while responses
to *adult female* instructions provide a standard for female mental health.

RESULTS

Table I presents the group mean and standard deviations within the Israeli
nonclient, client and therapist populations, as well as those of the American
therapists in the Maslin and Davis (1975) study, when these populations are
partitioned by rater's sex and ratee sex. While no main or interaction effects on
the Stereotype scores were found in either the nonclient or client populations,
significant main effects were obtained in the Israeli therapist population for
rater sex, $F(1,54) = 4.77, p < .033$ and ratee sex, $F(2,54) = 6.02, p < .004$. The

group means in Table I show that female therapists had more stereotypically masculine views of mental health than did male therapists for all categories, i.e., adult, male and female mental health. The main effect for ratee sex expressed itself in traditional sex-typed standards of mental health; the means (rater sex collapsed) for healthy adults (168.5) and healthy males (167.8) were similar and more toward the masculine pole than the mean for female mental health (158.0).

TABLE I

Means and standard deviations of Israeli nonclients, clients, and therapists vs. American Therapists (Maslin & Davis, 1975) partitioned as to sex on sex-stereotypic items

| | Ratee sex | | | | | |
| | Adult | | Male | | Female | |
	$\overline{X}$	SD	$\overline{X}$	SD	$\overline{X}$	SD
Israeli Ss						
Nonclients						
Male	171.9	8.5	170.5	11.3	167.5	21.2
Female	170.9	11.6	179.0	15.5	170.3	12.1
Clients						
Male	169.6	14.1	170.5	18.2	157.5	18.6
Female	168.9	19.1	170.3	15.8	164.4	16.8
Therapists						
Male	166.8	12.0	163.7	7.4	154.9	15.2
Female	170.3	11.5	172.0	7.0	161.2	8.3
American therapists						
(Maslin & Davis, 1975)						
Male	162.3	6.4	166.6	8.1	154.8	16.0
Female	162.4	7.0	166.7	8.4	166.4	11.0

The standard deviations in Table I reveal that the therapist population had the smallest variance in sex stereotype scores, followed by the nonclient and client populations. The mean standard deviations were 10.2, 13.3 and 17.1 for the therapist, nonclient, and client populations, respectively. Thus therapists had the highest degree of concordance with regard to sex-linked mental health standards, while clients manifested the widest range of disagreement. A Cochran's C test for homogeneity of variance in the nonclient, client, and therapist populations showed that these group differences in variance were significant at the .05 level.

Table I shows that male and female therapists in the Maslin and Davis (1975) study had almost identical standards of mental health for both adults and males. Male therapists, however, viewed female mental health as significantly more stereotypically feminine ($p < .01$) than did female therapists. Within-sex comparisons showed that female therapists did not perceive any significant differences between the healthy female and the healthy male or adult, while male therapists viewed female mental health as significantly more feminine than male mental health. Israeli female therapists, in contrast, perceived the healthy female as significantly more feminine than the healthy male, $t(18)$ = 2.97, $p < .01$, while there were no significant differences in male therapists' ratings of healthy female vs. healthy male or adult. Between-sex comparisons revealed that the only significant difference between the Israeli therapists was with regard to standards of male mental health, as female therapists maintained significantly more masculine standards for the healthy male than did male therapists, $t(18) = 2.42, p < .05$.

Planned comparisons were carried out to test for congruency of therapist-client stereotypes of mental health. Some interesting trends were observed even though none of the ts reached the .05 level of significance. Thus female therapists' perceptions of the healthy male, $\overline{X}$ = 172.0, were more congruent with those of male clients, $\overline{X}$ = 170.5, than were standards of male therapists, who perceived male mental health as more stereotypically feminine, $\overline{X}$ = 163.7. Similarly, female therapists' perceptions of female mental health, $\overline{X}$ = 161.2, were more congruent with those of female clients, $\overline{X}$ = 164.4, than were those of male therapists, $\overline{X}$ = 154.9, who also perceived the healthy female as being more stereotypically feminine.

DISCUSSION

Israeli female therapists of the present study held traditionally stereotypical perceptions of mental health and viewed the healthy female as significantly more feminine than the healthy male. Male therapists did not view female and male mental health as significantly different. These findings contradicted those of Maslin and Davis (1975), in which female therapists perceived the healthy female as similar to the healthy male, while male therapists maintained traditional stereotypically masculine and feminine standards of mental health. Because the present study replicated the instrumentation and instruction set of the Maslin and Davis study and the differences could not be attributed to differences in professional status or experience between samples, cultural factors may be responsible for these obtained differences. Thus while Israel ostensibly has an equalitarian, socialistic tradition and women serve alongside men in such diverse areas as the military, government and industry, it still tends to be relatively traditional in its outlook toward family, child upbringing, and the role of the sexes. While women often work because of economic necessity, they are employed largely in secondary service roles and devote their main psychological and physical efforts to children and family.

It is interesting to note that Israeli male therapists perceived male mental health as significantly more "feminine" than did female therapists. This sex difference in perception of male mental health is not replicated in the American studies of therapist sex-stereotypes (e.g., Broverman et al., 1970; Maslin & Davis, 1975), and we can only speculate as to why this difference occurs. The cultural norm for healthy males in the Israeli sample as a whole, $\overline{X}$ = 171.0, is more stereotypically masculine than that obtained in the Maslin and Davis (1975) study, $\overline{X}$ = 166.7. Our male therapists may be more sensitive, emotional, and nonaggressive as compared to the stereotype of masculinity in the general population and perhaps project these personal attributes on to their ratings of male mental health standards. Female therapists' standards of male mental health, on the other hand, may be more reflective of existing cultural norms and stereotypes as to what constitutes appropriate masculine behavior.

Of the three major populations the therapists were the only group in which a main effect was found for *ratee sex*. Thus therapists had the strongest sex-stereotypes of mental health and perceived healthy males and adults as alike and more masculine than healthy females. While there were similar trends in the client population, these trends did not reach statistical significance because the variance in this group was significantly larger than in the therapist population, which had the lowest variance of the three groups studied. Whether mental health professionals have more clearly defined standards of mental health than their clients and hence exhibit less variance in their ratings of healthy behavior or, alternatively, are employing rigid growth-prohibiting stereotypes of mental health can be resolved only by further research.

A related issue is that of congruency between therapists' and clients' perceptions of sex-appropriate behavior. Goldstein (1962), for example, has indicated that conflicting expectations of therapists and clients may negatively affect the therapeutic process. Thus sex biases or stereotypes that conflict with the client's aspirations may be counterproductive. It is interesting to note in this respect that the female therapists' standards for male mental health, in the present study, were more congruent with male clients' standards than were those of male therapists, who held relatively feminine standards of male mental health. Similarly, female therapists' standards for female mental health were more congruent with those of female clients than were standards of male therapists, who viewed the healthy female as more stereotypically feminine. The task force set up by the American Psychological Association in 1974 to study sex-biases in psychotherapy reported that female therapists are often discriminated against with male clients predominantly assigned to male therapists and women and children to female therapists. Our findings with regard to congruency of client-therapist mental health standards question the advisability of such assignment biases. Future studies should try to examine whether congruency of client-therapist sex based mental health standards indeed are related to improvement criteria in therapy.

Caution must be exercised in interpreting the above findings. Thus while sex role stereotyping exists as a general phenomenon, it is less clear that it systematically influences individual judgments of single patients. The problem with most of the research is that it deals with general stereotypes of the healthy adult, male or female or real or simulated clinical material about a male or female patient. Such studies call for an intellectual response and may not be representative of actual clinical intervention. Thus hypothetically a clinician may respond in a sexist fashion on an attitude questionnaire but not so in his/ her clinical work or alternatively be non-sexist on a questionnaire but behave in a sexist fashion in his/her therapeutic endeavors. The research of choice would require observation of the therapy process itself.

Steinmann (1974) in a series of cross-cultural studies found that women perceive themselves as balanced between orientation to self fulfillment and family values. However they perceive that men would prefer them to be much more strongly oriented towards the family and more passive than they perceive themselves. Steinmann in fact found that men wish women to be more balanced between self fulfillment and family values. Steinmann also found that male psychologists described the ideal women as more self oriented than the ideal woman of the national sample of women. These findings suggest that males in general as well as male therapists don't necessarily impose sexist notions on females in general since their ideal woman is much more self oriented than that of the national sample of women.

Billingsley (1977) found that male therapists chose significantly more feminine treatment goals for *all* their clients regardless of sex wheras female therapists chose significantly more masculine goals. It may be that therapists consider themselves to be atypical of their sex role stereotype and encourage the adoption of cross sex-role behavior in their clients. Therapists tended to respond to client's pathology rather than client's sex in formulating treatment goals. Thus therapists chose significantly more feminine treatment goals for explosive (psychotic) clients than for restricted (phobic) clients. There was no main effect for client sex nor did client sex interact with any other variable with regard to treatment goals.

In conclusion one must be cautious of generalizations such as that of the APA Task Force on Sex Bias and Sex Role Stereotyping in Psychotherapy that "psychologists expect women to be more passive and dependent than men". Such a "uniformity myth" based on general attitude questionnaires such as Broverman's, ignores the extreme variance of clinical work with individual clients. All patients are not the same nor are all therapists and hence conclusions should be stated in terms that respect differences. Viewing women as different from men is not enough. We have to also consider women at different age levels, different categories of pathology, socio-economic class differences, marital status and the like. We also must consider characteristics of therapists based on such demographic variables and their clinical interaction with different groups of women. These variables may contribute more to treatment variance than client's sex as Billingsley's (1974) study indicates. While stereotyping may occur with regard to general attitude objects such as "women" or "patients", it is least likely to occur when specific individuals are rated or treated.

Ben Gurion University of the Negev
and the Hebrew University of Jerusalem

REFERENCES

Billingsley, Donna
    1977 Sex bias in psychotherapy: an examination of the effects of client sex, client pathology and therapist sex on treatment planning. Journal of Consulting and Clinical Psychology 45: 250–256.
Broverman, I. K., Broverman, D. M., Clarkson, F. E., Rosenkrantz, P. S., and Vogel, S. R.
    1970 Sex role stereotypes and clinical judgments of mental health. Journal of Consulting and Clinical Psychology 34: 1–7.
Chesler, P.
    1972 Women and Madness. Garden City, N. Y.: Doubleday.
Deutsch, C., and Gilbert, L.
    1976 Sex role stereotypes: Effect on perceptions of self and others and on personal adjustment. Journal of Counseling Psychology 23: 373–379.
Epstein, C. F.
    1970 Woman's place: Options and limits in professional careers. Berkeley: University of California Press.
Goldstein, A. P.
    1962 Therapist-patient expectancies in psychotherapy. New York: Macmillan.
Horner, M. S.
    1969 Sex differences in achievement motivation and performance in competitive and non-competitive situations. (Doctoral dissertation, University of Michigan, 1968). Dissertation Abstracts Interantional 30: 407B. University Microfilms No. 69–12: 135.
Kravetz, D.
    1976 Sex role concepts of women. Journal of Consulting and Clinical Psychology 44: 437–443.
Maslin, A., and Davis, J.
    1975 Sex role stereotyping as a factor in mental health standards among counselors-in-training. Journal of Counseling Psychology 22: 87–91.
Report of the task force on sex bias and sex role stereotyping in psychotherapeutic practice
    1975 American Psychologist 30: 1169–1175.
Rosenkrantz, P., Vogel, S., Bee, H., Broverman, I., and Broverman, D.
    1968 Sex role stereotypes and self-concepts in college students. Journal of Consulting and Clinical Psychology 32: 287–295.
Steinmann, A.
    1974 Cultural values, female role expectancies and therapeutic goals: Research and interpretation. In V. Franks & V. Burtle (eds.), Women in Therapy. New York: Brunner/Mazel.

I. KALLAB, Ph.D., J. ABU NASR, Ph.D., and I. LORFING, M.A.

SEX ROLE IMAGES IN LEBANESE TEXT BOOKS*

SUMMARY. Previous research in socialization indicates that sex role definitions in a certain society are internalized and learned by its members through different means among which are books. The present study examines the image of women and the sex roles attributed to them in 52 Arabic text books printed between 1970–1977 and are currently in use by the majority of elementary and intermediate schools in Lebanon. The results of this survey are consistent with previous research findings on French, American and Italian books, which depict women in the traditional role of mother, whose major function is cooking and housekeeping. They are presented as martyrs who may only attain self-fulfillment through sacrificing their life for their husbands and children.

INTRODUCTION

The concepts of masculinity and feminity have been given serious attention in recent literature. This interest, which was an outgrowth of the women's movement, has focused attention on sex role stereotypes and their potential adverse effect on personality development. The exploration of the socialization process, through which sex-typing behavior is learned, has become a challenge to social scientists in different parts of the world.

Research in socialization indicates that sex role definitions in a certain society are internalized and learned by its members. According to the social learning theory sex-typed behavior is mostly acquired through "observational learning" or "identification". "Observational learning behavior" Mischel contends, "may result from watching what others (models) do, or from attending to symbols such as words and pictures." Mischel 1970, 29). It is through observational learning that the young child acquires the role of male or female and the characteristics ascribed to it. Mischel goes on to say, "Undoubtedly, TV, movies, books, stories and other symbolic media play an important part in transmission of information about sex-typed behavior and the diverse consequences to which they may lead when displayed by males and females." (Mischel, 1970, 45).

Based on the assumption that books are a good vehicle for introducing models to children, it is imperative that we become aware of the types of models that are being advocated in their books through the written word and through illustrations. This paper is an attempt to investigate the image of women and the sex roles attributed to them in Arabic children's text books.

Studies in the U.S.A. by Weitzman et al. (1972), and Stewig and Higgs (1973), in France by Bereaud (1975) and Chombart de Lauwe (1971), in Italy by Belotti (1975) report identical results. Women in American, Italian and French books are depicted as mothers and housewives whose major task is cooking and keeping everybody happy. They are characterized by passivity,

I. Gross, J. Downing, and A. d'Heurle (eds.), Sex Role Attitudes and Cultural Change, 131–140.
Copyright © 1982 by D. Reidel Publishing Company.

dependence, and submission. Generally they are left out of the labor market and are assigned home related roles. One may conclude that women in the majority of French, American and Italian books are presented in rigid stereotype sex roles. Bereaud contends that in French books the traditional notion of women's roles "persist despite changed realities" (Bereaud 1975, 195). Chow (1976) who studied Chinese picture books indicates that sex role differentiation in these books is less marked than that of American or French ones. The roles attributed to women in Chinese books are more in line with the real situation in China than the American, French or Italian books, which do not reflect the real image of women in their respective countries.

METHOD

Sample

The present study examines the image of women and the sex roles attributed to them in Arabic text books used in the elementary and intermediate schools in Lebanon. Lebanon is a country of about 2.5 million people with approximately 4000 elementary and intermediate schools representing a mosaic of religious and ethnic groups. Fifty two Arabic textbooks printed between 1970–1977 and are widely in use, comprised the sample of this study. The general topics include: Arabic Readers, Conversation, Grammar, Civic Education, Take-home exercise books, School exercise books and Teacher's Guide.

The authors of the books represent the different religious groups in the country. The content differs theoretically from one book to the next, but in reality many of the texts are identical in style, in terminology, in imagery and in pattern. We feel that we can assert with confidence that our findings are applicable to other Arabic textbooks which were not included in this study, based on the repetitive pattern we encountered in the books reviewed.

The 52 books selected were read word for word and the vocabulary, idioms and images pertaining to females were recorded. The analytical framework was designed to include the following areas: female sex roles, identity, sex role traits, functions and status.

All these conceptual areas were operationally defined and data were then exposed to quantitative and qualitative analysis. The study was divided into two parts, one dealing with the written text, and the other with the illustrations that supplement it. In this presentation we will restrict our discussion to the written word only.

RESULTS

Women's Roles

Data in Table I depict traditional and stereotyped sex roles assigned to women.

It is evident that the most frequent role attributed to females is that of mother (45%). Next in importance, judging by the frequency of its occurrence (27%), is the "little girl" who is being prepared for motherhood. Grandmother, who has served her term and is passing on the torch to the next generation, occupies third position in this hierarchy (14%). The working woman, who does not venture too far from the domestic arena, is occasionally assigned to service jobs similar to her home responsibilities as nursing, housekeeping dressmaking and baking. Other roles include wife, lady of leisure, fantasy women, aunts, cousins, and neighbors.

TABLE I

Female sex roles in Arabic textbooks

	No.	Percentage
Mother	325	45
Grandmother	104	15
Little Girl	190	27
Working Woman	39	5
Others	57	8

Identity

Women's identity as revealed through her name, her age and physical characteristics attributed to her appears in Table II. It is clear from these data that mother's identity as an individual is not a necessity. The mother appears as a symbol rather than a person. She is identified by her role as mother. No personal name is given to her, but she is known by her oldest son's name, which is a common practice in Lebanon. Her physical attributes and her age are completely ignored.

TABLE II

Female identity in Arabic textbooks

	Mother		Grandmother		Little Girl	
	No.	%	No.	%	No.	%
Physical attributes	1	5	52	63	10	12
Age	1	5	28	34	52	61
Personal name	–	–	–	–	23	27
Named by sons	19	90	2	3	–	–

Modesty of women in the traditional Arab Islamic culture has been reported by Antoun (1968), Hilal (1971), Youssef (1978), Dodd (1973) to be extremely important for family status. To ensure "modesty", society has "effective institutional mechanisms that preclude women's contact with the opposite sex; to mention only a few; sex segregation in public and private schools, rigid sex segregation at work, and informal separation of the sexes in most recreational and often familial activities." Youssef (1978, 78). Beck and Keddie (1978) and Hilal (1971) contend that the treatment of women as a person centers on her sexual role; therefore confining her to her home and keeping her anonymous becomes necessary to protect her "modesty" and family honor.

Grandmothers also appear as anonymous except in a few cases where they are identified by their oldest son's name. Their identification by the role they occupy is predominant. Grandmother's physical appearance, which is consistent in all textbooks, is clearly defined as a seventy-year old who has been ravaged by years.

The little girl in most instances is given an Arabic name which does not have a religious connotation. She is referred to occasionally as "little mother" and is seen always at home. Her age is between six and ten, a safe age to write about since she can still play with boys.

There is more freedom to talk about little girls and grandmothers, since they do not represent a threat to family honor. Little girls do not menstruate and grandmothers have reached menopause and hence are not sexual beings (Beck and Keddie 1978).

Sex Role Traits

Stereotyped female-traits were also apparent throughout the literature. A number of traits attributed to the mother, the grandmother and the little girl were identified.

Mother is presented as tender, protective, loving, neat, always busy in house chores, a good cook, a good hostess, a shrewd bargainer, and a dependent individual. In the relationship to her children she is characterized as overprotective while with her husband she is submissive and dependent. The most outstanding trait of all mothers, however, is martyrdom where the theme is repeated 105 times. Children are burdened with feelings of gratitude, expressed on mother's day in stale adult language which is remote from the world of childhood. In the traditional code of "modesty" Hilal (1971) and Chamoun (1967, 1974) have stated that women are expected to be "self-denying" and their feminity is synonymous with self-effacement. This attitude may be true of the majority of mothers in Lebanon today, although one may detect some change among young mothers. Statistical evidence to support this observation is lacking.

The grandmother is characterized by weakness, nurturance, tenderness and lack of skill in house chores as a result of old age; nevertheless, she is presented as continuously active. Economically, grandmother is dependent on her son with whom she generally lives, which is an acceptable practice in Lebanon. Her relationship with the children is warm, protective and loving.

The little girl is described as kind, obedient, well mannered, quiet, clean, polite, dependent, passive, helpless and cries easily. In a few instances she is frivolous and insists on having new clothes. She is sensitive to the beauty of nature and likes flowers.

Sex Role Functions

Data in Table III summarize the traditional sex role functions performed by females and the frequency of their occurance. Chamoun (1974) reports that the image of the Lebanese woman is that of an eternal mother whose main role as a wife is to reproduce, feed and protect her children. This image is reflected in the data where 34% of such references are made to her presence in the kitchen and the dining room. The amazing thing is her ability to manage all these meals skillfully alone, along with all the other house chores without showing any signs of fatigue or boredom.

TABLE III
Female functions in Arabic textbooks

	Mother		Grandmother		Little Girl	
	No.	%	No.	%	No.	%
Cook & feeder	65	34	15	13	14	16
Housekeeper	25	13	15	13	31	34
Purchaser	16	8	–	–	–	–
Disciplinarian/						
Child protector	60	32	30	27	30	34
Educator – Relating						
tales	–	–	33	29	–	–
Other	24	13	20	18	14	16

Spending a lot of time in the kitchen is generally true of most Lebanese women, but this pattern is gradually changing with more females seeking outside employment, especially in Beirut. Housekeeping is another time and energy consuming task which the mother is reported to perform without complaining or tiring. Dress making, knitting, crocheting, and attending to a sick child are given equal distribution. Many of these tasks are still performed by women with the exception of dress making, which is not a necessity any more since ready-made clothes are available and dress makers are abundant.

The purchasing mother is also included but her buying responsibilities are limited to the purchase of vegetables and fruit for cooking and textiles for sewing. It is interesting to note that from the roaming vendor who comes to her door step, she buys her vegetables and fruit alone, while she is accompanied by one of the children to go to the textile shop downtown.

Child care is one other major responsibility delegated solely to the mother where she is mainly concerned with the child's physical and emotional well being to the point of overprotection. Thirty two percent of the references are concerned with child care and discipline. Discipline is used by mothers to instill in the child the acceptable social values of obedience, cleanliness, neatness, health care, respect to father and guests and proper behavior with siblings. The disciplinary measures used by mothers vary from mild, looking at a child disapprovingly, to harsh by scolding and screaming.

The functions of the grandmother are limited to helping the mother in housekeeping, relating tales and historical events to grandchildren, and mediating to protect the children from father's wrath and harsh discipline. Being the father's mother, she can exert this influence on him while his wife cannot, nor can she use the same measures with the daughter-in-law. The children in turn love and respect her.

The little girl is being trained at an early age for her role as mother in the traditional meaning of the word. "Little mother" practices all the tasks that her mother does in cooking, housekeeping and attending to younger siblings. She takes care of brothers at home, younger or older, but the functions are reversed outside the home where the brother, younger or older, is supposed to protect his sister. For her leisure time the only toy she owns is a doll which is meant to prepare her for the role of motherhood as well.

The most significant finding was the fact that no mother in these references had a job or a profession. Motherhood is presented as a full time, life time job. Three generations, mother, grandmother and child are all playing the role of mother. This finding is in line with studies reported earlier on American, French and Italian books but it does not reflect the image of the Lebanese woman today.

In the last decade, due to the impact of modernization, Lebanon has seen profound changes in the different socio-economic and political institutions. The rates of change, however, have been uneven between different sections of society with respect to urbanization and modernization. As a consequence, female roles and statuses in Lebanon today vary greatly by age, education, social class and geographic location (Prothro & Diab 1974).

One of the most obvious changes is the access of education to women. In 1970, women represented 23% of the student enrollment in universities while, in the total Lebanese population aged over 25, 18% were university graduates. Here again we should stress the rural-urban differentials (UNESCO 1974).

Outside employment of women is becoming an economic necessity for Lebanese families. A report by the Ministry of Planning (1972) and Lebanese Family Planning Association (1974), based on data collected in 1970, have indicated that 9% of married women are working on different levels of employment ranging from 17% professionals to 21% skilled workers, 17% clerks, 17% industrial workers and other professions. We expect this number to have increased considerably as a result of the war where more women have become bread earners of their families. We have no data so far to substantiate our observations.

Studies on attitudes towards working women reveal a positive change of attitude to outside employment among the younger generation of middle-class wives as reported by Prothro & Diab (1974) and Accad-Sursock (1974).The national survey of the Ministry of Planning (1972) has indicated that 18% of the total female population were employed, 34% of whom were professionals, 10% office employees, 19% industrial workers, 26% domestic workers and 23% in agriculture. The textbooks, nevertheless, continue to present the traditional role of Lebanese women, which may still be prevalent in remote rural areas and among the lower class sector of society (Prothro & Diab 1974, Antoun 1968).

The danger here lies in perpetuating the status quo and reinforcing the traditional sex role by providing stereotype models for behavior which are likely to be internalized by readers who are repeatedly exposed to these models. Thus through observation of the same sex traditional model the young child soon acquires the role ascribed to him or her as a male or female.

Status

A closer look at the roles assigned to women in the textbooks as mother, grandmother and little girl and the functions they perform in their respective roles, reveals the traditional outlook toward women in the Arab Moslem culture where her status is derived only from marriage and motherhood. Her world is the "domestic world" and almost all her activities are carried out within the limits of the house (Beck and Keddie 1978). It is interesting to note that her image in western books, where the Christian culture is predominant, is not much different.

Restricting women's activities to the menial domestic tasks where she is not required to make any decisions or even share in making them may be considered an evidence of her low status profile in the family structure. Other indices of low status may be her exclusion from intellectual endeavours, from the labor market and from participation in cultural, educational, social or voluntary activities.

The women's total economic dependence on the male as husband or son is one other evidence of her low status. She is described as being always a consumer of goods and never a producer. Even as a consumer her decisions are limited and remain within the domain of the household as cook and dressmaker thus suggesting her inferior ability in decision-making on issues other than food and clothing.

The working woman is also restricted to her domestic service role which is menial and less respectful. Agricultural work, housekeeping, dressmaking, or nursing are professions that have a low status profile in the social scale. To the male are left those tasks that require more intellectual ability, thus depicting his superior status.

As wife, the texts reviewed do not give any clue to her status. This has been completely neglected and left out of the literature. She is mentioned only once as a wife disciplining the children to provide an atmosphere where their father can concentrate on his work.

CONCLUSION

The image of women reflected in 52 Arabic textbooks, which comprised the sample of this study is consistent with the traditional portrait which appears in French, American and Italian books. She is a full time, life time mother whose major functions are cooking and housekeeping. The women and the little girl have no identity of their own. They are presented as martyrs who may attain self-fulfillment only through sacrificing their life for their husbands and children.

Little girls have nothing to aspire to other than being mothers in the traditional sense. Their future occupational world centers around the kitchen and the dining room. Sex traits are stereotyped and rigid to the point of stifling any imagination or creativity on the part of the little girl whose life has been mapped out for her.

A new outlook in children's Arabic textbooks is necessary, especially after the war where women and men are equally responsible for rebuilding the new Lebanon. With the tremendous changes that have occured in the country, women's roles are bound to be modified to meet the new challenge. Women in Lebanon today are doing more things than housekeeping and cooking. They are attending universities, entering the labor market as directors, artists, professionals, writers, journalists; they are very active in voluntary work and they are also voting and driving cars. The textbooks should reflect the image of educated women, career women, and the partnership in a marriage relationship rather than the dichotomy now presented.

The social values of unquestionable obedience, dependence, submission and passivity, all characteristics of a weak personality attributed to women, should be replaced by new values that reveal strength of character, creativity and independence. These traits are essential if women are to be partners in the process of development.

Books are good vehicles for learning and therefore they should be used to extend the horizons of children rather than limit their imagination with prescribed roles. Adult characters as models in books could be influential in altering the traditional images of women. They could serve as a catalyst that would inspire women to more dynamic roles. Hilal (1971) asserts that the masculinity and feminity concepts belong to the realm of culture and are subject to change. With that hopeful note, our plea goes to writers of children's books to incorporate models that may inspire little girls to more creative dynamic roles as women and little boys to more realistic roles as men.

Beirut University College

NOTE

* This research was funded by the Institute for Women's Studies in the Arab World through a grant from the Ford Foundation.

REFERENCES

Accad-Sursock, R.
    1974 La femme Libanaise: de la tradition à la modernité. Travaux et Jours 52: 17–
       38.
Antoun, R. T.
    1968 On the modesty of women in Arab Muslim villages: A study in the accommoda-
       tion of traditions. American Anthropologist 70: 671–697.
Beck, L., and Keddie, N.
    1978 Women in the Muslim World. Cambridge, Massachusetts: Harvard University
       Press.
Belotti, E. G.
    1975 Du côté des petites filles. Paris: Éditions de femmes.
Bereaud, S. R.
    1975 Sex role images in French children's books. Journal of Marriage and the Family,
       February: 194–207.
Chamoun, M.
    1967 Problèmes de la famille au Liban. Travaux et Jours 25: 13–40.
Chamoun, M.
    1974 Couples. Travaux et Jours 52: 5–14.
Chombard de Lauwe, M. J.
    1971 Image de soi et images culturelles de l'enfant. Psychologie Francaise 16(3–4):
       185–198.
Chow, E. N. L.
    1976 Sex role images in children's picture books: China, France and the United States.
       Paper presented at the 71st Annual meeting of the American Sociological Associa-
       tion, New York.
Dodd, P.
    1973 Family Honor and the forces of change in Arab society. International Journal of
       Middle East Studies 4: 40–54.
Falconnet, G., and Lefaucheur, N.
    1975 La Fabrication des Mâles. Vienne: Seuil.
Hilal, J.
    1971 The management of male dominance in 'traditional' Arab culture: A tentative
       model. Civilization 21(1): 85–95.
Lebanese Family Planning Association
    1974 The Family in Lebanon, Beirut, Vol. 1.
Le Nouvel Observateur
    1976 Special Famille, Novembre 8.
L'Express
    1979 Papa Fume et Maman Lave, March 10: 43.
Prothro, E., and Diab, L.
    1974 Changing Family Patterns in the Arab East. Beirut, Lebanon: American University
       of Beirut.
République Libanaise, Ministère du Plan Direction Centrale de la Statistique
    1972 L'Enqûete par sondage sur la population active au Liban. Beirut, 1: 144–
       145.
Stewig, J., and Higgs, M.
    1973 Girls grow up to be momies: A study of sexism in children's literature. School
       Library Journal 98: 44–49.
United Nations, Economic and Social Council
    1974 Études sur les relations existante entre les possibilités d'education et les possibilités
       d'emploi offertes aux femmes au Liban. Paris.

Weitzman, L. J., Gifler, D., Hokada, E., and Ross, C.
    1972 Sex role socialization in picture books for preschool children. American Journal
         of Sociology 77(6): 1125–1149.
Youssef, N.
    1978 Status and fertility patterns of Muslim women. Women in the Muslim World. In
         L. Beck and N. Keddie (ed.), Cambridge, Mass.: Harvard University Press.

RAMA S. PANDEY, Ph.D.

STRATEGIES OF HEALTHY SEX ROLE DEVELOPMENT IN MODERNIZED INDIA*

SUMMARY. Social modernity is defined by a coherent set of such variables as high achievement orientation, participative decision-making and broad human concern. It is measured by the range of these options available to men and women in different life sectors such as marriage, education and occupation. The present study is designed to identify the role of fathers and mothers in the socialization of adolescent boys and girls in social modernity and to analyze policy implications for healthy sex role development. Nine hundred parents in nine regions of India were interviewed to study marital, educational and occupational options open to them and to their adolescents. Four patterns were identified: the modernized pattern with high options, the traditional pattern with low options and transitional patterns (2) with mixed options. A dynamic policy is suggested to promote healthy sex role development in four patterns.

INTRODUCTION

Social modernity has been defined by a coherent set of variables such as high achievement orientation in education and occupation, participative decision-making and broad human concern. For systematic studies on the syndrome of social modernity, I would refer to Lerner (1958), McClelland (1961), Hagen (1962), Bellah (1965), Kahl (1968), Inkeles (1974), Doob (1967), Rogers (1969), Armer and Schnaiberg (1972) and Portes (1973). Lerner (1958), McClelland (1961), Hagen (1962), Inkeles (1978) and other scholars have studied national differences on individual social modernity. Safilios-Rothschild (1970) has concluded that a society is higher on modernity if it actually offers these options to all individuals and groups regardless of their age, sex, race or religion. Social modernity is also measured by the range of options open to individuals in different life sectors such as marriage, education and occupation.

A number of studies have focused upon sex role options in social change and modernization. These studies deal with sex role options of men and women and their impact on sex role socialization of boys and girls. Holter (1971), Safilios-Rothschild (1975), Haavio-Mannila (1975), Mednic (1975), Hareven (1975) and other scholars have studied recent changes in the sex roles of men and women and their links with changing social structure, particularly in social production, political participation, access to education and other social systems. Their participation in larger social systems defines their status and roles in family relationships. However, modernization affects men and women differently. Safilios-Rothschild (1978) finds that in practically all countries, working wives seem to be penalized by a transition that allows them to participate in the economic sector without corresponding changes being made in sex role stereotypes and role redefinitions that would allow their husbands to share with their

141

I. Gross, J. Downing, and A. d'Heurle (eds.), Sex Role Attitudes and Cultural Change, 141–149.
Copyright © 1982 by D. Reidel Publishing Company.

household responsibilities. According to Clausen (1978), studies in U.S.A. bearing directly on sex-differentiated responses of fathers or of either parent toward older children are relatively rare. Some recent cross-cultural studies, however, have found sex of parents and adolescent children as intervening variables in their social modernity. For example, Rosen (1962) has found that protective mothers and authoritarian fathers are significantly more responsible for the markedly low achievement motivation of boys in Brazil. Klineberg (1973), in his study of Tunisian adolescents, has concluded that sex and age have different effects on "attitudinal modernity" of their adolescent boys and girls. Cunningham (1972) has found that separation of both parents and students by sex shows significant correlations between students and parents of the same sex. Suzman (1973) has found early experiences more closely associated with modernity among females. This effect is most marked among women who were not working or who had never worked. Portes (1973) has identified intrafamily orientations as an important dimension of social modernity. This is defined by positive attitudes towards women's work outside home, the belief that women should make decisions independently from husbands and the belief that parents should take into account children's opinion.

Some studies on socialization of children in India have also supported the sex role distinction. Gore (1975) has concluded that the great educational gap between husbands and wives still continues for the society as a whole, but among those who have practiced white collar occupations for two generations or more, this gap has been considerably reduced. In a subsequent study (1977), he has identified increasing differences in occupation, education and age of marriage. He says that the age of marriage of the urban middle class has gone up largely because the future economic standing of a young boy depends upon his education. The rise in the age of marriage has meant that the girls have to be kept occupied during the years prior to marriage. Education provides the substitute occupation. The later age of marriage and education prior to marriage in case of girls raises problems for the joint family. Pandey (1975), in a study of youth in India, has found that parents and youth have high educational and occupational aspirations. However, the rural youth like to prepare women for feminine roles while the urban youth prepare for self-fulfillment. Both groups stress home science content for women's education.

These studies suggest sex role as an important variable in the social modernity of parents and children. Safilios-Rothschild (1975) has identified certain in- dicators of sex role options in social modernity. These options are related to marriage, education and occupation. The indicators of marital choices are identified here as (1) to marry or not to marry; (2) to marry with anyone regard- less of age, race, class, caste or religion; (3) to bear or not to bear children. The indicators of educational choices include (4) to go to school; (5) to pursue one's studies and graduate at college or professional school level. The occupa- tional choices are measured by (6) to work or not to work; (7) to work in a particular field; and (8) to work when single or married. This paper will focus upon these basic choices; whether these are available to both sexes of parents in modernized India; whether they offer these choices to their adolescent boys and girls; and how these choices are interrelated with each other in the socialization process. It will further analyze the policy strategies of healthy sex development in a modernized context. The paper will address the question of where in the social structure, actions toward change should be directed to promote healthy sex role development.

METHOD

Sample

A national sample of 816 families in India was selected on the basis of five criteria: regional subculture, rural-urban location, religion, income and family structure. It was assumed that these criteria represented socio-economic and cultural variations in the total population. The sample included approximately 100 families from each of the nine regions of India, and each regional subsample included families belonging to rural-urban locations, the four major religions of India, different income levels and joint/nuclear family types. Weight was given to minority groups and communities in order to project variations in attitudes and behaviors.

Instruments

An interview schedule was used to record the modernized background of parents and their child socialization practices. The first part of the interview schedule was addressed to the mother, and the second part to the father. The schedule was designed to collect data pertaining to economic and family background of parents and major systems of behavior that are covered under child socialization. These behavioral systems include feeding, training, parental relationship, play, schooling, housework, marriage and vocational preparation (Whiting and Child, 1953.). The interview schedule focused upon child socialization practices in traditional/modern dimensions. It included questions that elicited information on whether individual parents had strong achievement drive in feeding, training, schooling, and so forth, of their boys and girls; whether the parents involved their children in decision-making about their schooling, marriage, vocational preparation; and whether the parents provided children with a role model for developing concern for other human beings. A number of questions in two parts of the schedule were duplicated to elicit responses of both mothers and fathers in relation to the socialization of boys and girls. This paper will analyze the data pertaining to both sexes of parents and adolescents in three sectors of life: marriage, education and occupation.

RESULTS

The data are organized in four domains: (1) parents' background; (2) achievement orientation; (3) participative decision-making; and (4) human concern. The inclusion of variables in particular domains is based on the assumption that there is a unidimensional relationship between two variables, and particular variables are the best measurements of the domain in which they are included. To determine the amount of overlap between the variables of different domains, the technique of simultaneous canonical correlation has been used. According to Horst (1961), it yields the maximum correlation between linear functions of sets of variables.

The canonical correlations of the first four roots and their labels are given in Table I. The correlations of sex-linked variables pertaining to basic choices of individual parents and adolescent children are also reported. These choices are related to marriage, education and occupation. These indicate what mothers and fathers have for themselves and what they provide for their adolescent boys and girls. These choices are identified along three dimensions of social modernity: achievement orientation, participative decision-making and human concern.

These results show that in all three sectors of life – education, marriage and vocation – fathers' and mothers' background and child socialization practices are characterized by high options in the modernized pattern, low options in the traditional pattern and mixed options in the transitional patterns. However, some of their correlations indicate sex differences. In parents' backgrounds, mothers' occupation and women's status and roles (domain I) are such variables. In child socialization practices, vocational prospects and marriage perparation (domain II), handling of school problems (domain III) and marriage problems (domain IV) are other sex-biased variables. Modernized parents and their socializees have low options on these variables while parents and their children in other patterns, particularly in transitional ones, indicate high options. These transitional parents and their children have high options on certain other variables such as fathers marriage age (domain I), children's new ideas (domain II), school failure (domain III) and concerns for son's marriage (domain IV). These variables in four different patterns indicate strategies of healthy sex role development in modernized India.

POLICY IMPLICATIONS

The four patterns of social modernity in sex role development suggest social policy development in three sectors of life: marriage, education and occupation. A dynamic policy is required in increase options to both sexes of parents and their children in different patterns: modernized, traditional and transitional I and II. The marital strategy in the modernized pattern would focus upon changing the status and roles of women as wife and socializer and improving parents' orientations towards children's marriage preparation. The educational strategy

TABLE I

Simultaneous canonical correlations and loadings on first four roots (N = 816)

(.3 as cut off value)

DOMAIN & VARIABLES	Modern- ized Pattern	Tradi- tional Pattern	Transi- tional Pattern I	Transi- tional Pattern II
	I .764	II .499	III .461	IV .423
I. PARENTS' BACKGROUND				
Mother's education	.804			
Father's education	.706			
Mother's occupation			.538	
Mother's age at marriage (M)	.598			
Mother's age at first pregnancy (M)	.449			
Mother's work experience (M)			.510	
Mother's marriage type (M)	.362			
Concept of good wife (M)				−.445
Handling marriage problem (M)				.332
Concept of good husband (M)				.393
Family planning understanding (M)	.467	−.361		
Age of father's marriage (F)	.496			.480
Father's job movement (F)	.394			
Family planning understanding (F)	.365			
Participation in housework (F)		.344	.305	
Opinion about breadwinning and cooking		.366		
Opinion about women's status (F)			.351	.328
Feeling about marriage (F)			.337	
II. ACHIEVEMENT ORIENTATION				
Schooling				
School selection consids. (M)	.392			
Children asking questions (M)	.487			
Special help in education (M)	.665			
Educational achievements (M)	.461			
Reaction to failure, daughter (M)	.309			
Imp. of educ., son & daughter (M)	.551			
Managing girls' education (M)	.508			
Managing boys' education (M)	.534			
Educ. expectation from son (F)	.347			
Choice of fields, son (F)	.366			
Choice of fields, daughter (F)	.369			
Educ. consid. daughter (F)	.318		.308	
Reaction to new ideas (M)	.481			
Reaction to new ideas (F)	.317		.360	

Table I (continued)

DOMAIN & VARIABLES	Modern-ized Pattern	Tradi-tional Pattern	Transi-tional Pattern I	Transi-tional Pattern II
	I	II	III	IV
	.764	.499	.461	.423
Vocational preparation				
Preparing daughter for job (M)	.470			
Age, self-supporting, daughter (M)	.316			
Opinion, job training, daughter (F)	.401			
Response to expectation from son (F)		−.314		
Prospects for daughter (F)		.317		
Marriage preparation				
Marriage preparation, duaghter (M)		−.377		
Sex education, topics (M)			−.445	
Sex educ. desirable, son & dgtr. (F)	.390			

III. PARTICIPATIVE DECISION MAKING

Schooling				
Reasons for son's school performance (M)			.328	
Reasons for daughter's school performance (M)			.336	
Difference over daughter's education (M)	−.308			
Exam. Failure, son (M)				.343
Exam. Failure, daughter (M)				.336
Vocational Preparation				
Vocational decisions for son (F)	.313			
Vocational decisions for daughter (F)	.315			.310
Marriage Preparation				
Marital choice for son, daughter (M)	.625			
Premarital social contacts, son (M)	.554			
Marriage type preferred (M)	.590			
Acutal marriage decisions, son (F)	.408	−.483		
Actual marriage decision, daughter (F)	.393	−.474		
Premarital social contact, son (F)	.419	−.366		

Table I (continued)

DOMAIN & VARIABLES	Modern- ized Pattern	Tradi- tional Pattern	Transi- tional Pattern I	Transi- tional Pattern II
	I	II	III	IV
	.764	.499	.461	.423
IV. HUMAN CONCERN				
Marriage Preparation				
Marriageable age of son (M)	.515			
Marriageable age of daughter (M)	.612			
Response of adolescents (F)				.317
Marriageable age of son (F)	.387			.371
Marriageable age of daughter (F)	.393			
Marriage considerations for son (F)	.315			.406
Marriage considerations for daughter (F)	.472			
Marriage problems with daughter (F)			−.373	

M = Mother respondent
F = Father respondent

would enhance parents' ability to deal with their children's schooling problems. The occupational strategy may upgrade the occupational status of mother in the socialization process and improves job prospects of boys and girls. These policies may be promoted by consciousness raising of the father and mother and through necessary institutional changes. In the past three decades, several social legislations have been passed in India to raise the status and roles of women and children and to increase their social options. It appears, however, that these policy changes do not deeply impact on the attitudes and values of the people, even in the modernized sector of the population. The other three patterns of child socialization would require a broader policy intervention into the parents' background and their child socialization practices for healthy sex role development.

University of Minnesota — Duluth

NOTE

* This paper is based on my study of child socialization in India. For full details of the study, see Pandey, R. S. (1977), *Child Socialization in Modernization*, Bombay, India: Somaiya Publications.

REFERENCES

Armer, N. and Schnaiberg, A.
   1972 Measuring individual modernity. American Sociological Review: 301–316.
Bellah, R. N.
   1965 Religion and Progress in Modern Asia. New York: The Free Press.
Clausen, J. A.
   1978 American research on the family and socialization. Children Today: 7–10.
Cunningham, I.
   1973 The relationship between modernity of students in a Puerto Rican high school
         and their academic performance, peers and parents. International Journal of
         Comparative Sociology: 203–220.
Doob, L. W.
   1967 Scales for assaying psychological modernization in Africa. Public Opinion Quar-
         terly: 414–421.
Gore, M. S.
   1977 Familial change and the process of socialization in India. Paper presented at the
         Study Group meeting of the International Association for Child Psychiatry and
         Allied Professions.
Gore, M. S.
   1975 Indian Youth: Processes of Socialization. (Manuscript)
Hagen, E. E.
   1962 On the Theory of Social Change: How Economic Growth Begins. Homeswood,
         Illinois: The Dorsey Press.
Haavio-Mannila, E.
   1975 Convergences between East and West: Tradition and Modernity in sex roles in
         Sweden, Finland, and the Soviet Union. Women and Achievement. New York:
         John Wiley, pp. 71–84.
Hareven, T. K.
   1976 Modernization and family history: Perspective on social change. Signs: 190–
         206.
Holter, H.
   1975 Social roles and social change. Women and Achievement. New York: John Wiley,
         pp. 6–19.
Horst, P.
   1961 Generalized canonical correlations and their application to experimental data.
         Journal of Clinical Psychology No. 14.
Inkeles, A.
   1978 National differences in individual modernity. Comparative Studies in Sociology:
         47–72.
Kahl, J. A.
   1958 The Measurement of Modernism: A Study of Value in Brazil and Mexico. Austin:
         University of Texas Press.
Klineberg, S. L.
   1973 Parents, schools and modernity: An exploratory investigation of sex differences
         in the attitudinal development of Tunisian adolescents. International Journal
         of Comparative Sociology: 221–244.
Lerner, D.
   1958 The Passing of Traditional Society: Modernizing the Middle East. New York:
         The Free Press.
McClelland, D. C.
   1961 The Achieving Society. Princeton, N. J.: Van Nostrand Co.

Mednic, M. T. S.
  1975 Social change and sex role inertia. Women and Achievement. New York: John
        Wiley: 85–103.
Pandey, R.
  1975 India's Youth at the Crossroads. Varanasi, India: Vani Vihar.
Pandey, R. S.
  1977 Child Socialization in Modernization. Bombay, India: Somaiya Publications.
Portes, A.
  1973 The factorial structure of modernity: Empirical replications and a critique.
        American Journal of Sociology: 15–44.
Rogers, E. M.
  1969 Modernization Among Peasants. New York: Holt, Rinehart and Winston.
Rosen, B. S.
  1962 Socialization and achievement motivation in Brazil. American Sociological Review:
        612–624.
Safilios-Rothschild, C.
  1978 Trends in family: A cross-cultural perspective. Children Today: 38–45.
Safilios-Rothschild, C.
  1975 A cross-cultural examination of women's marital educational and occupational
        options. Women and Achievement. New York: John Wiley: 48–70.
Safilios-Rothschild, C.
  1970 Toward a cross-cultural conceptualization of modernization. Journal of Compara-
        tive Family Studies No. 1.
Smith, D. and Inkeles, A.
  1974 Becoming Modern: Individual Change in Six Developing Countries. Cambridge,
        Massachusetts: Harvard University Press.
Suzman, R. M.
  1973 Psychological modernity. International Journal of Comparative Sociology: 273–
        287.
Whiting, J. W. H. and Child, I. L.
  1953 Child Training and Personality: A Cross-Cultural Study. New Haven: Yale Uni-
        versity Press.

DENIS CHIMAEZE UGWUEGBU, Ph.D.

EFFECTIVENESS OF SELF-PERSUASION IN PRODUCING HEALTHY ATTITUDES TOWARDS POLYGYNY

SUMMARY. Western-educated Nigerian men and women tend to develop close mindedness to polygyny with severe social and psychological consequences, if there was need for them to be involved in polygynous marriage. The present research attempted to produce tolerance to polygyny in educated Nigerians through the technique of improvisation. The subjects were 95 students who either wrote or did not write pro-polygyny essays. Half of the essay and non-essay groups were pretested. The subjects rated some items that measure attitude to polygyny. The results showed that improvisation led to pro-polygyny attitude. It was concluded that improvisation technique could serve as an effective means of preparing Nigerians to be more open minded enough to perceive polygyny as a legitimate family role any Nigerian could play.

INTRODUCTION

Traditional African cultures and values are being eroded by contact with Western-type education. One traditional cultural practice which has met with increased rejection among educated Africans is probably polygyny.

Among the Africans the traditional objective of marriage is procreation. A childless marriage or a marriage without a male child is deemed a failure. A husband is, therefore socially and morally expected to marry more wives to off-set the "abnormality" in his family.

Educated Africans tend to reject the traditional beliefs and values associated with the practice of polygyny. The rejection creates stress and conflict between such a western-socialized African and his environment. Family conflicts in literate homes over compliance with traditional prescriptions for polygyny or western proscriptions against polygynous behaviour often lead to divorce. The initial depressive shock and other family conflicts brought about by the idea of a second wife in the family could be reduced through a programme of attitude change. The general purpose of the research reported in this article was to produce positive attitude toward polygyny through the use of improvised role-playing.

Research employing improvisation techniques to produce attitude change is non-existent in Nigeria. However, in the western world, a body of research in attitude change evidences a strong support for improvisation as the most reliable technique in producing attitude change (Zimbardo & Ebbesen, 1970). The effects of improvisation in attitude change has been detailed by Janis and King (1954), King and Janis (1956), and Watts (1967). Generally, the objective of improvisation is to make a stimulus person more tolerant of a given contrary position by having him explicitly espouse a set of opinions which are contrary to his initial position. In other words the subject is led to take a critical look at

151

I. Gross, J. Downing, and A. d'Heurle (eds.), Sex Role Attitudes and Cultural Change, 151–155.
Copyright © 1982 *by D. Reidel Publishing Company.*

his/her position and to persuade himself/herself of a counter-norm position. If the subject is successful in the self persuasion through improvisation of a counter-attitudinal argument, a movement toward positive attitudinal direction may occur.

The present report describes an attempt to produce among educated Nigerians a positive attitude toward polygyny, through improvised counter attitudinal essay writing. It was expected that the subjects who improvised essays in favour of polygyny would show more positive attitudes toward polygyny than those who did not improvise any essay. In line with this theoretical expectation three hypotheses were tested in the study: (1) Subjects who espoused positive opinions about polygyny through essay writing should express more tolerance for polygyny than those who did not improvise essays. (2) Subjects who were sensitized by pretesting should evidence greater attitude change to polygyny than those who were unpretested. (3) A two-way interaction effect of essay and testing was also expected.

METHOD

Sample

Ninety-five University of Ibadan undergraduates from the Faculty of the Social Sciences, who were taking various psychology classes, participated in the study. The fewness of female students (a total of 11 females) who participated in the experiment prevented the inclusion of sex as a factor in this study. The subjects participated in the experiment under laboratory conditions.

Procedure

Solomon's (1949) 4-Group Design was used. When the subjects arrived for the experiment, they were randomly assigned to any of the four groups designated as groups A, B, C and D. Group A rated a 4-item questionnaire, entitled 'A Survey of Marriage Attitudes', and after that they wrote a 30 minutes essay in favour of polygyny. Four outline arguments in favour of polygyny were made available to the subjects as a guide for their improvised essays: (1) Polygyny is an aspect of unique African culture. (2) The concept of marriage in Africa is to have children. Men are socially expected to have children. (3) African men are by nature polygynous. (4) The percentage population of marriageable women is greater than that of men. The improvised essay was followed immediately by a second rating of the 4-item questionnaire.

Group B rated the questionnaire twice with an interval of about 30 minutes between the first and the second ratings. Group B did not write any essay. Group C improvised an essay in favour of polygyny, using the same outline as group A, and then rated the questionnaire while group D rated the survey of marriage attitude questionnaire only once without improvising any essay.

Two independent variables (Essay versus Testing) each with two levels (improvised essay vs no-essay X pretested versus unpretested) yielded a 2 X 2 design. The questionnaire items of interest scored by the subjects are listed below: (1) The practice of monogyny is against the African culture. (2) A husband should marry more than one wife if he has the money. (3) Government should make laws against polygyny. (4) The Nigerian man is by nature polygynous.

The items were a 7-step Likert-type scale. With the exception of item 3 which was reversed all the other items ranged from Agree Definitely = 1 to Disagree Definitely = 7, with the mid-point of the scale anchored Neither Agree-nor-Disagree = 4. The subjects were assembled and debriefed at the conclusion of the study.

RESULTS

The subjects' responses from the post-test scores were subjected to a 2 X 2 ANOVA (Campbell & Stanley, 1967). The results indicated significant main effects of essay on two items and of testing on the other two.

Item 1 (The practice of monogyny is against the African cculture), indicated a significant main effect of pretesting, $F(1, 94) = 4.10, p < .05$. The mean values for the main effect showed that the pretested group disagreed more $(\overline{X} = 4.12)$ with the item than the unpretested group, $(\overline{X} = 3.10)$. In like manner, item 2 (A man should marry more than one wife if he has money) showed that the pretested group disagreed more $(\overline{X} = 4.79$ versus 3.65) with the statement than the unpretested group, $F(1, 94) = 7.5, p < .01$. For items 1 and 2 the subjects who were unsensitized by pretesting tended to be more pro-polygyny than the pretested group. The finding lends some support to the second hypothesis of the study.

"Government should make laws against polygyny" (item 3), and "the Nigerian man is by nature polygynous" (item 4) each indicated a significant main effect of improvisation, $F(1, 94) = 14.5, p < .001$ and $F(1, 94) = 12.8, p < .001$ respectively. Examination of the mean values for item 3 indicated that those who improvised essays in favour of polygyny disagreed more than the non-essay group that government should make laws against polygyny $(\overline{X} = 2.5$ versus $\overline{X} = 4.0)$. The subjects who improvised essays also agreed more $(\overline{X} = 3.3)$, than the non-essay group $(\overline{X} = 4.7)$, that the Nigerian man is by nature polygynous. The data which showed significant main effects for improvisation lent some support to hypothesis 1 in the present study. Surprisingly there was no interaction effect as was predicted.

Finally a comparison was made between the index scores of pre- and post-ratings of subjects in group A as well as those in group B to examine whether there was any change in scores. A t-test of dependent measures indicated a significant effect for group A $t(1) = 9.32, p < .05$, or a significant pro-attitude toward polygyny as a result of the essay. The analysis for the B group did not approach significance.

DISCUSSION

The predicted interaction effect between essay and testing was not realized. However, the expected main effects of testing and improvisation received some support. Subjects who improvised a counter-attitudinal essay were more pro-polygyny on two items than those who did not improvise essays. Two others (items 1 & 2) indicated the main effects of testing. The direction of the mean values showed that the subjects who were unsensitized by pretesting were more pro-polygyny than those who were sensitized by pretesting. In other words pretesting tended to produce biasing effects against polygyny in the subjects' ratings.

Improvisation was more effective for two items on our questionnaire than testing, while testing was more effective on the other two items than improvisation. Such a discrepancy is due to item-type differences. Theoretical explanation for the item-type discrepancies is offered by Zimbardo and Ebbesen (1970). According to Zimbardo and Ebbesen statements or items that are informationally or factually based are more effective in producing improvisation effects while items that are "self-relevant" or self-descriptions of the subjects' expectations or feelings are less effective in producing attitude change due to self-persuasion. In the present study item 2 could be classified as a self-relevant statement, items 3 and 4 as factually based statements while item 1 seems not to fit into any of Zimbardo and Ebbesen's classifications.

Generally, minimum support was found for improvisation. What is important, however, is the cross-cultural significance of the superiority of improvisation over non-improvisation group among Nigerian University students in those items that are factually based. Western religious upbringing of many of these students makes the idea of polygyny highly unacceptable at this stage of these young Nigerians' lives. Since most of them are forward looking, they are not yet perceptible to those societal demands on couples without children or with the "wrong" sexed children. However, the technique of improvisation was sufficiently sensitive enough to produce positive attitude change towards polygyny.

Positive attitude or "open mindedness" to polygyny would allow an individual Nigerian man and woman to accept a second wife in the family should circumstances demand it. Such open mindedness achieved through improvisation would protect a wife and husband from family conflicts, frustrations, and divorce that usually result from the presence of a second woman in the home of an educated Nigerian family.

University of Ibadan

REFERENCES

Campbell, D. T., and Stanley, J. C.
    1967 Experimental and quasi-experimental designs for research. Chicago: Rand McNally
          & Co., p. 25.

Janis, I. L., and King, B. T.
1954 The influence of role-playing on opinion change. Journal of Abnormal and Social Psychology 49: 211–218.

King, B. T. and Janis, I. L.
1956 Comparison of the effectiveness of improvised versus non-improvised role-playing in producing opinion changes. Human Relations 9: 177–186.

Solomon, R. L.
1949 An extension of control group design. Psychological Bulletin 46: 137–150.

Watts, W.
1967 Relative persistence of opinion change induced by active compared to passive participation. Journal of Personality and Social Psychology 5: 4–15.

Zimbardo, P. and Ebbesen, E. B.
1970 Influencing Attitudes and Changing Behavior. Reading, Mass: Addison-Wesley Publishing Co., pp. 56–57.

P. NIEMELÄ, Ph.D.

OVEREMPHASIS OF MOTHER ROLE AND INFLEXIBILITY OF ROLES

SUMMARY. Data about overemphasis of the mother role from several of the author's own studies are reconsidered. Overemphasis of the mother role is related to inflexibility of different female roles in present society. For women with a developed personal identity, overemphasis of the mother role is considered to be related to unaccepted ambivalence about motherhood, and suggestions are made how to support psychological work during life transitions related to the mother role. Overemphasis of the mother role for women with a less developed sense of personal identity, low self-esteem and incapability for adequate interpersonal relationships is understood as a necessary defense which should not be undermined as it supports these women and makes them capable of functioning normally, although in a restricted way, among other people.

A Woman Has Many Roles

Finnish society is one where a woman has good opportunities for education and for working outside the home. Therefore she has many roles. She is a worker, a sexual partner, a life companion, a mother. She often experiences conflicts between her roles. She can resolve her role conflicts in several ways. Some women can recognize a conflict, feel it, work it through and possibly solve it so that they accept their different needs but cope with the conflict. Others are unable to come to a flexible solution and overemphasize one of the roles. In this paper I am going to report some of my group's results related to overemphasis of the mother role.

The Studies Referred To:

The first is the Longitudinal Study (Heino 1978, Hiiri and Koski 1977, Uusitalo 1975, Waenerberg 1979), in which we interviewed and tested 38 women at the end of their first pregnancy as well as one, two, three and four years after the birth of the child, in order to describe the effects of how a future mother works through her role conflicts and difficulties concerning motherhood.

The second is the Housewife Study (Anias-Tanner and Wälimäki), where we interviewed 30 housewives whose youngest child had recently entered school, in order to describe how a mother changes her roles and subidentities when her children are growing independent.

In the third study on Female Identity (Kallio and Lahtinen 1977) we interviewed all of the 48 women between 30 to 40 years old who were living in a middle class suburb, in order to study the emphasis of different female roles in the age period when a woman's feminine identity can be considered fully developed and the woman is not yet confronted by the role changes of old age.

157

I. Gross, J. Downing, and A. d'Heurle (eds.), Sex Role Attitudes and Cultural Change, 157–162.

All the women interviewed are psychiatrically healthy and living in normal life conditions. The interviews took on average about three or four hours. The students and research workers were trained for the interviews. The results mentioned below are tested with the analysis of variance and are statistically significant.

Overemphasis of Mother Role Compared to Other Role Emphasis

In the female identity study we compared women emphasizing a mother role, a partner role and a worker role. The women who overemphasize their mother role see themselves, their marital relationships and their activities more negatively than do women who overemphasize their role as a partner or as a worker. The different aspects of life were experienced most positively by the women who did not emphasize any particular role. The overemphasis of one role, and particularly the emphasis of the mother role, seems to be, for a woman, an unhealthy attitude towards feminine roles.

Measuring Overemphasis of Mother Role

The scale to measure the overemphasis of mother role was developed in the Longitudinal Study. A factor analysis describing conscious attitudes towards motherhood produced as a second factor a cluster of statements given below, with factor loadings in parenthesis:
— Joy of motherhood can only be felt by a woman who herself has given birth (.775)
  — Every woman should experience childbirth at least once in her life (.741)
  — A woman can really feel herself a woman only after giving birth (.688)
  — Pregnancy and childbirth make a woman a real woman (.680)
  — I believe motherhood will be the happiest thing in my life (.438)
Agreement with each statement was measured on a five point scale, and the estimates were summed for each subject. The data from the Longitudinal Study show that five women emphasized motherhood very much and about half at least somewhat. Mothers who agree with this scale in pregnancy, agree significantly more so several years later, too.

Ideal Mother and Self Image as a Mother

Data from all three studies show that mothers who overemphasize motherhood also conceptualize the Ideal Mother as one who Forgets Her Own Needs (unselfish, selfsacrificing, adapts her life to the child), Forgets Her Own Feelings (patient, never feels annoyed with the child, never resents child care) and Aims To Be a Perfect Mother. The mothers with this mother ideal also report themselves to be closer to this mother ideal than do other mothers.

Mothers Who Overemphasize the Mother Role as Mothers

As reported in Niemelä (1977, 1978) the Longitudinal Study shows that mothers emphasizing motherhood had, compared to other mothers of the study, more painful deliveries with more tenseness and less cooperation with midwives. They felt themselves more insecure in nursing, with more ambivalent feelings towards the baby. They experienced breast feeding as more unpleasant and breast fed a shorter time. With the growing child they still had more ambivalent feelings, were more binding towards the child as well as more possessive and overprotective. They act in an inadequate way on the child's terms, help the child when it does not need help and reward a clinging contact from the child. The children of these mothers, when they are two and three years old, are more restless and less positive and cooperative towards the tester. They also have a more clinging contact with the tester and they are less enterprising. In a doll test they distance themselves more from the mother figure than do other children. The mothers who emphasize the mother role are obviously more inadequate as mothers.

The Unaccepted Ambivalence for Motherhood and Role Conflicts

Through many studies (e.g., Bibring 1961, LeMasters 1957, Niemelä 1977) we know that becoming a mother is a major life transition in a woman's life. A future mother encounters many conflicts between her roles. The unresolved conflicts reflect themselves in her ambivalence towards her pregnancy and motherhood. Resolving these conflicts presumes that a future mother can approach, accept and work through her ambivalent feelings about pregnancy and motherhood and the conflicts related to her roles and relationships.

Women who overemphasize motherhood cannot approach and accept their ambivalent feelings, because their image of an ideal mother excludes acceptance of these very feelings. Instead, we may understand the overemphasis of motherhood as an armour against these ambivalent feelings, which prevents working out conflicts about becoming a mother. Similarly mothers who must redefine their roles as their children grow have to approach and work on their difficult feelings about motherhood. Our Housewife Study shows that mothers who overemphasize the mother role cannot carry out this psychological task but are bound to their earlier significance as a mother.

Can We Develop a Healthy Attitude Towards the Mother Role?

If we consider overemphasis of mother role due to untreated role conflicts and ambivalence about becoming a mother, then future mothers should be given support in this difficult emotional work. The staff at the maternal clinics and in maternal hospitals should be educated to encourage mothers to talk about their insecurities and role conflicts.

For three years I have led small groups where future mothers (and couples) can discuss their difficulties from midpregnancy to some months after childbirth. Although I do not yet have any hard data about differences between this group and the control group, I can already say that participants have experienced these discussion groups as helpful for working out ambivalence and role conflicts about parenthood. I would think that these groups have helped many mothers to avoid overemphasis of the mother role. However, in these groups I have met mothers who deny all their ambivalence and idealize motherhood, despite the groups' support for psychological work. Who are these mothers and can they be helped?

Overemphasis of Mother Role and Low Self Esteem

The data from the Longitudinal Study show that idealizing mothers are younger and have less education than the other mothers of the study. Erik H. Erikson (1968) has emphasized that the formation of personal identity continues far into the twenties. Education and working experience also help to give a feeling of personal identity and self esteem. It is possible that some women seek the mother role in order to be somebody and to find their identity through motherhood.

According to the Female Identity Study data the women who emphasize the mother role also have a weaker sense of feminine identity. They experience their bodies as less attractive and their character as more submissive than do other women. The mothers in the Longitudinal Study who emphasize the mother role actually report that motherhood is important for them in order to feel themselves women. The overemphasis of the mother role may be understood as a way of coping with a fragile self-esteem as a person and as a woman.

Overemphasis of the Mother Role and Inadequate Human Relationships

Women who overemphasize the mother role, both in the Longitudinal Study and in the Female Identity Study, report that they are less satisfied in their marital and sexual relationships. The women in the latter study report that they experience the marital relationship mainly as a family and less as a relationship between a woman and a man. This study also shows that these mothers feel the meaning of a child in a woman's life as less important than do other mothers. To them the husband and the children mean less as human relationships.

The Object Relation Technique (1955) data from the Longitudinal Study show that these mothers are generally more insecure, inadequate and distant in relationships with other people. According to these data they are less capable of intimate interaction in their marital relationships. They are less able to be genuinely concerned about other people. Instead they are more possessive and binding. These women are less capable of forming satisfying human relationships. It may be that these women seek motherhood in order to find their place and function among other people through the mother role. They therefore define their relationship with their husbands in terms of a family rather than as an intimate relationship. They therefore also emphasize their own role as a mother more than their relationship with their children.

Overemphasis of the Mother Role is a Coping Mechanism

These mothers whose identity and interpersonal relationships are fragile obviously need their defense of overemphasizing the mother role. Without it these women would function worse, also as mothers. We all agree that it is better for a child to be overprotected than to be treated insecurely and inconsequently.

Stereotyped overemphasis of motherhood is here understood as a necessary defense against low self-esteem resulting in dysfunction. This defense may also be understood as a result of the mother's personality and life situation rather than a cause of inability to cope with role conflicts and insecurities in interpersonal relationships. Therefore, group discussions which encourage the more healthy mothers to work out their role conflicts, must not take away this defense from less healthy mothers.

We may understand roles as analogous to psychological defense and coping mechanisms. These are many and various. Some of them are on a high level, are flexible and allow and encourage a person to act in an adequate way in a given situation. Others are more rigid, more stereotyped, making a person act always in the same restricted way. A mother who overemphasizes her role as a mother, acts in this role also in her work or when with her husband or friends. How can we encourage her into more flexible roles?

University of Turku

ACKNOWLEDGMENT

The research reported in this paper was made possible by the financial support of the Social Science Committee, Finnish Academy of Science, and by research grants from Aaltonen and Wihuri foundations.

REFERENCES

Anias-Tanner, H. and Wälimäki, H.
  1977 Kotiäidin identiteetin uudelleenmäärittelyprosessi nuorimman lapsen kouluun-menovaiheessa. Unpublished M. A. thesis in Psychology, University of Turku, Finland.
Bibring, G. L.
  1961 A study of the psychological processes in pregnancy and of the earliest mother-child relationship. In Eissler, R. S. (ed.), The Psychoanalytic Study of the Child. London: The Hogarth Press.
Erikson, E. H.
  1968 Identity, Youth and Crisis. London: Faber and Faber.

Heino, L.
  1978 Valmentautumisen ja raskauden aikaisten asenteiden yhteys synnytyksen hallintaan ja synnytyskokemukseen. Unpublished M. A. thesis in Psychology, University of Turku, Finland.
Hiiri, S. and Koski, A.
  1977 Kaksi vuotiaan lapsen emotionaalinen käyttäytyminen suhteessa siihen, miten äiti hyväksyy ja kokee äitiytensä. An unpublished M. A. thesis in Psychology, University of Turku, Finland.
Kallio, K. and Lahtinen, H.
  1977 Heikon ja vahvan identiteetin kuvaaminen 30—40 vuotiailla naisilla. An unpublished M. A. thesis in Psychology, University of Turku, Finland.
Le Masters, E. E.
  1957 Parenthood as crisis. Marriage and Family Living 19: 352—355.
Niemelä, P.
  1977 Psychological preparation for parenthood. Paper presented at the fifth international congress of Psychosomatic Obstetrics and Gynaecology, Rome.
Niemelä, P.
  1978 Idealizing motherhood. Paper presented at the Sex Role Convention of the International Council of Psychologists, Oslo.
Uusitalo, R.
  1975 Odottavan äidin tiedostettu ja tiedostamaton raskauden ja äitiyden hyväksyminen. An unpublished M. A. thesis in Psychology, University of Turku, Finland.
Waenerberg, P.
  1979 Lapsen hoidon ja imetyksen suhde äitiyden hyväksymiseen. An unpublished M. A. thesis in Psychology, University of Turku, Finland.

SUSAN BRAM, Ph.D.

SEX WITHOUT REPRODUCTION: VOLUNTARY CHILDLESSNESS AS A RESPONSE TO CONTEMPORARY SEX ROLES

ABSTRACT. Voluntary childlessness is examined in an attempt to investigate alternatives to traditional sex role patterns. A comparative study of childless couples compared to those who delay and those who are parents is reported. Interview data from both husbands and wives is utilized. The childless are discovered to be white, educated middle class couples primarily of Protestant backgrounds, currently nonreligious. There are some indications that the wife experienced her family of origin as tense and attributed this to children; otherwise, family background is not a differentiating factor. The childless lifestyle is characterized by the themes of individualism and nontraditional sex roles: the wives are more involved in work and achievement, the men tend to be more creative and less traditional in their work plans. The marriages of the childless are more egalitarian and companionate as measured by household tasks arrangements. There is more emphasis on personal growth within the marriage. A discussion of the implications of the childless data focuses on the problems in the modern organization of parenthood and on the intrinsic contradictions in modern sex role definitions, especially for the woman.

The question posed for the conference – "How can we develop healthy attitudes toward masculine and feminine roles?" – is indeed a complex one. In order to give a full answer to such a question we need to consider several related issues, such as "How are masculine and feminine roles defined today?", "Are these sex roles changeable or immutable?", and "Are there alternatives to these sex roles?".

In this paper we will address the latter question by examining data on a group of people who have chosen an alternative to traditional sex role definitions in their own lives – the voluntarily childless. This group is of both theoretical and practical interest to our conference. The theoretical importance of childlessness is that in many respects it represents the antithesis of traditional sex roles, especially for women. Because the childless have chosen to live out their sexual lives without utilizing their reproductive potential, they are eliminating what many believe to be the basis for biological, psychological and social sex role differentiation. Although researchers differ in the importance they place on the reproductive function in understanding sex differences, there is no question that in modern western society parenthood is organized in such a way as to differentially affect males and females. Women who have chosen not to become mothers are *de facto* testing the assumption that women are different from men because of their participation in childbearing and related functions (childrearing, socialization of the young); both men and women who forego parenthood are experimenting with the limits of their own sex role identities. Thus, an understanding of how the childless live gives us insight into the range of possible sex role behaviors, at least within a heterosexual pairing, and can provide a

163

I. Gross, J. Downing, and A. d'Heurle (eds.), Sex Role Attitudes and Cultural Change, 163–175.
Copyright © 1982 *by D. Reidel Publishing Company.*

challenge to many traditional assumptions about sex role behavior and gender identity.

The study of childlessness is of practical importance as well. As we have discussed elsewhere (Bram, 1978), childlessness itself is a social indicator of changed attitudes towards parenthood, fertility, sexuality and the family. Because of their "deviant" position in society the childless are astute observers of the social realities and offer an articulate critique of modern parenthood and how it is arranged. Furthermore, a review of their lifestyle, especially over time, provides a comparison group for longitudinal studies of so-called "normal" adult development and marital relationships. In our role as helping professional it is of particular importance that we develop as diversified a view of human potential as possible in order to offer the fullest range of choices to others.

As recently as seven years ago, when we were conducting our first study on voluntary childlessness (Bram, 1974), there was little interest in the topic among social scientists or the public and most people viewed the childless as social or psychological deviates. Since that time, however, increasing rates of childless-ness, spurred on by major social developments, such as the greater educational and economic participation of women, have caused a recognition of the impor-tance of this phenomenon and a reexamination of the view of childlessness as pathological.

Developments on the policy level in the United States (e.g., the Supreme Court ruling on abortion, support for the ERA, funding for family planning) have gone hand in hand with changes in fertility attitudes and behavior among men and women, especially in the younger cohorts. Age-specific birth rates in the United States reached low levels in 1974 and 1975 as family size decreased and rates of childlessness increased. Although the overall rates of childlessness in the U.S. are still low — it is estimated that about 7% of evermarried women age 45–49 are childless (U.S. Bureau of the Census, 1976) — the proportion who are childless among married women age 15–29 has been increasing since the 1940 birth cohort, challenging previous demographic forecasts. For example, between 1960 and 1974 the percentage of evermarried women age 20–24 who remained childless rose by 2/3, from 24.4% to 40.6%, and for women age 25–29 the increase was close to 60%, from 12.6% to 19.6% (U.S. Bureau of the Census, 1975; Van Dusen & Sheldon, 1976). Overall birth expectations for wives 18–29 have decreased as well — the percentage of women in that age group expecting no children increased from 3.1% in 1967 to 4.6% in 1975 (U.S. Bureau of the Census, 1976). Social surveys in the U.S. and Western Europe continue to find higher than predicted percentages choosing childlessness, especially, but not only, among the college-educated (Blake, 1974; Gerson, 1977; Hoffman, 1974; Niphuis-Nell, 1976; Pohlman, 1974; Rozeboom, 1974; Veenhoven, 1974). Popular literature reflects this trend as well (Peck and Senderowitz, 1974; Whelan, 1975).

In a recent article on the future of marriage and family in the United States, Westoff (1978) states that "If current first-order birth rates were to continue, about 30% of women would never have any children, an unprecedented, but not totally implausible development". (p. 81) Although, as the U.S. Bureau of the Census said in 1971, "It is too early to say if these trends foretell a future increase in the proportion of women remaining childless, or merely a pattern of later childbearing", (p. 160) it is evident that changes are occurring in fertility attitudes and behavior and, we believe, these in turn reflect changes in attitudes toward sex roles.

With the new interest in the topic of childlessness there has been a recent growth in the number of exploratory studies in the United States and Western Europe (den Bandt, in progress; Gustavus and Henley, 1971; Houseknecht, 1977; Nason and Poloma, 1976; Ory, 1978; Silka and Kiesler, 1977; Thoen, 1977; Veevers, 1973, 1976), utilizing a variety of methodologies and sampling techniques. Despite the diversity of approaches, there has been a striking convergence of findings among these studies. Here it will suffice to report our own study results and refer to other studies only where their findings diverge significantly.

METHODS

Sample: The sample was composed of 83 white educated middle-class couples chosen systematically from married students' housing in a small midwestern city in the United States.[1] Of the sample 30 couples were determined to be voluntarily childless, 29 delays, and 24 parents, with the age, marital duration, and employment status reported in Table I.

Instrument: A lengthy in-depth interview schedule composed of closed and open-ended questions was utilized to investigate family background, history of the fertility decision, attitudes toward parenthood and children,[2] individual lifestyle, marriage pattern, social life and social pressures. Husband and wife were interviewed in their home by male and female interviewers respectively, at the same time but in separate rooms to facilitate independent responses.

Analysis: Data on the three groups were analysed separately for husbands and wives, utilizing chi-square or analysis of variance statistics. (Only a portion of the data will be presented here.)

RESULTS

Background: The childless are white, educated, middle-class couples in their mid-20's, married an average of 3—4 years. They tend to be of Protestant background

TABLE I

Length of marriage; age of wives and husbands; employment status of wives and husbands, for total sample, childless, delays, and parents

	Total Sample	Childless	Delays	Parents
Length of Marriage n.s.	3.54	4.06	3.00	3.54
Age of Wives p < .05 F = 4.167	25.32	26.53	24.66	24.63
Age of Husbands n.s.	26.36	27.43	25.63	25.81
Employment Status of Wives				
Homemaker	8	1	1	6
Employed	51	19	21	11
Student	24	10	7	7
Total	83	30	29	24

$p < .02$
$\chi^2 = 12.31$, df = 4

	Total Sample	Childless	Delays	Parents
Employment Status of Husbands				
Employed	37	22	8	7
Student	42	8	19	15
Total	79	30	27	22

$p < .01$
$\chi^2 = 12.66$, df = 2

but currently non-religious. The women are slightly more likely than the delays or parents to be first born or only children of nontraditional (educated and/or working) mothers. The women view their parents' marriage as unhappy and attribute this problem to children. Otherwise, family size and family background as measured in this study do not differentiate the childless from the delays or parents. About 40% of the childless women and 10% of the men state that they had decided to remain childless prior to marriage; the rest decided later, following periods of vacillation and postponement. There are several indicators that the decision was more important to the woman than the man. For example, she has given it more thought and lists more reasons for the decision.

Motivations: The childless value many of the same aspects of children as do the delays and parents, and there is agreement on some of the costs of children. The values and costs mentioned by a majority of all three groups of men and women are listed in Table II. Although the childless value these aspects of children,

TABLE II

Consensual values and costs of children: Categories chosen by a majority of childless, delays and parents as 'very' or 'somewhat' important

Values of Children	
1. Affiliation	Primary ties and affection, e.g., gaining a sense of family, sharing new experiences with spouse, having a new source of companionship and affection.
2. Stimulation and Novelty	Watching a growing child.
3. Achievement	Helping a child to develop into a healthy human being; the sense of accomplishment.
4. Power and Influence	Wanting to influence another human being; to have an impact on the world.

Costs of Children
1. Overpopulation
2. Interference with Wife's Education
3. Loss of Freedom in the Marriage

they hope to attain them through alternate means, e.g., teaching, counseling. In contrast, they perceive more costs of children than do the others and weight them more strongly in their lives. The costs mentioned significantly more often by the childless men and women are in Tables III and IV.

TABLE III

Chi-square analyses of costs of children that differentiate childless wives from delays and parents

Cost of Children & Item		Childless (n=30)	Delay (n=29)	Parent (n=24)	Significance
1. PSYCHOLOGICAL COSTS					
"Not sure I'd make	V*	46.7	13.8	12.5	$p < .05$
a good parent."	S	23.3	34.5	25.0	
	N	30.0	51.7	62.5	
"Don't like the	V	56.6	17.3	12.5	$p < .01$
responsibility."	S	36.7	31.0	20.8	
	N	6.7	51.7	66.7	

Table III (continued)

Cost of Children & Item		Childless (n=30)	Delay (n=29)	Parent (n=24)	Significance
2. ACHIEVEMENT COSTS					
"My work is more	V	60.0	6.9	16.7	$p < .01$
important than	S	20.0	20.7	8.3	
children."	N	20.0	72.4	75.0	
3. INTERFERENCE WITH LIFESTYLE					
"Want freedom to	V	83.4	31.0	25.0	$p < .01$
do things spon-	S	13.3	34.5	29.2	
taneously with	N	3.3	34.5	45.8	
my spouse."					
4. INTERFERENCE WITH MARRIAGE					
"My spouse and I	V	30.0	6.9	4.2	$p < .01$
are too close to	S	40.0	27.6	4.2	
spend time with	N	30.0	65.5	91.6	
a child."					

* Note: All subjects responded to all items. A separate chi-square analysis was performed for each item. The numbers refer to the percentage in each group who rated the item as "very", "somewhat", or "not" important in their thinking about having children.

TABLE IV

Chi-square analysis of costs of children that differentiate childless husbands from delays and parents

Cost of Children & Item		Childless (n=30)	Delay (n=29)	Parent (n=24)	Significance
1. FINANCIAL STRAIN					
"Would rather spend	V*	16.7	3.7	4.5	$p < .05$
my money on other	S	40.0	18.5	18.2	
things."	N	43.3	77.8	77.3	
2. PERSONAL RESPONSIBILITY					
"Don't like the	V	43.3	11.1	9.0	$p < .01$
responsibility."	S	33.3	37.0	27.4	
	N	23.4	51.9	63.6	

* Note: All subjects responded to all items. A separate chi-square analysis was performed for each item. The numbers refer to the percentage in each group who related the item as "very", "somewhat", or "not" important in their thinking about having children.

Individual lifestyle & marriage patterns: Measures of the individual lifestyle of the childless men and women included questions on daily activities, sources of satisfaction and dissatisfaction in life, personal values, goals for the future and self-image. In general, the childless were found to differ from the delays and parents in two major respects. They were found to be *more individualistic*, concerned with attaining particular life goals, and were *less traditional* in their sex role definitions. Their highly idiosyncratic lifestyle is based on spontaneity and freedom — they value the opportunity to engage in leisure time pursuits as they wish and to pursue achievement goals at their own tempo.

Their tendency to deviate from the traditional sex role definitions is particularly evident in their attitudes toward work. Both spouses mention achievement goals as a major source of satisfaction in life. The childless women, however, are more likely to be employed than the parents and are more likely to be employed fulltime in professional jobs than either the delays or parents. They place a greater value on work in their lives and are more likely to mention achievement goals as a current source of satisfaction and a desire for the future. A small, but significant portion of the men deviate from traditional male career paths in their choice of creative work, such as photography or painting, and some plan to stop supporting themselves in the future.

In terms of self-image and personal values, the childless women and men differ from the others in some important respects. The childless wives are significantly more likely than the other women to rate themselves as dominant on a self-rating scale, and less likely to rate themselves as dependent. The childless men are less likely than the others to rate themselves as occupationally competitive or dominant. In addition, both men and women are more supportive of women's liberation movement values, such as equal independence training for men and women, and equal responsibility for housekeeping and childcare, than are the other groups.

The childless marriage is consistent with the lifestyle values. On measures of decisionmaking and division of household labor, the childless were found to be significantly more *egalitarian and companionate*. These findings were maintained even when the data were analysed with a control for wife's employment, suggesting that the equal participation of the childless wife is not merely a function of her employment status. The childless also place more emphasis on *personal growth* in the marriage. For example, they speak of marriage as a source of independence and identity.

SUMMARY

The childless described here are white middle class educated young adults who have decided relatively early in their lives and marriage that having children and becoming parents is not for them.[3] Although the women give some indication of possible origins of this decision in their recollections of family life, the primary motivating factors appear to have arisen from experiences and observations as adults.

An examination of the motives for childlessness in itself provides a critique of the institution of parenthood as it is currently organized in our society. Of note is the fact that, in line with our introductory statements, it is parenthood, not children, that the childless wish to avoid. The childless are as likely to choose childlessness for proactive reasons — things they want to do which would be interrupted by parenthood, as for reactive reasons — things they don't like about having children. This suggests that the choice to remain childless is more than just a refusal to accept an adult role in society.

Both spouses recognize that parenthood as it is currently defined has more of an impact on the woman's life choice than the man's; thus, both male and female include the wife's educational and career goals among their reasons for childlessness. That the issue of childbearing is more conflictual for the woman is indicated by her emphasis on psychological costs — anxiety and interference with personal growth. This probably reflects both the concerns with achievement and affiliation discussed below, as well as the tensions associated in contemporary society with the high standards for performance of mothering functions. In addition, there is strong evidence that the childless men also desire to free themselves from the constraints of parental responsibility that fatherhood carries in our society.

Two major motives emerge in the analysis of the decision to remain childless — achievement and affiliation. Both the men and the women feel that parenthood would conflict with individual achievement goals that they value. They are also concerned with the conflict between the demands of parenthood and the affiliative bonds of the marriage. They recognize that another member in the family would interfere with their lifestyle and might disrupt the marital dyad. Some also voice the fear that the tendency for women to carry the burden of childcare (all best intentions aside) could easily diminish the egalitarianism in the marriage. Thus, the lifestyle and the marriage pattern highly valued by the childless would be threatened by parenthood.

The lifestyle of the childless reflects their attempt to combine the achievement and affiliative motives within a framework that is mutually satisfying to the spouses. It appears that a requisite to meeting this goal is a willingness to defy traditional sex role definitions. Although the manner in which the couples combine these needs varies greatly within the sample, some general characteristics are evident.

(a) The childless women place more value and energy on their work roles than do the others, even though they are not always career-oriented.

(b) The men are equally or less involved in their work than their wives and in some cases deviate from the traditional male work pattern by choosing creative pursuits or depending on their wives for financial support.

(c) The childless perceive themselves as nontraditional and are willing to express their nontraditional values in regard to sex roles, such as equal household and economic participation of the sexes.

(d) They manifest these values in their arrangement of married life. Their division of labor and decisionmaking in the home are significantly more egalitarian than the other groups.

It is of note that the childless stand apart from both the delays and parents in their tendencies to share work and leisure within the marriage. That even the delays were less egalitarian than the childless suggests that not having children is not sufficient to create an egalitarian marriage. One must not have children and not have the mental disposition towards having children in order to develop these characteristics. These findings lead us to conclude that the childless lifestyle is different, not only because of the structural components of the situation, i.e., the employed wife, the absence of children in the home, but also because of a value orientation of the childless toward equal participation of the sexes and toward self-actualization.

DISCUSSION

Our study, as well as the subsequent research and survey data, clearly indicates that voluntary childlessness is an emerging alternative to traditional sex role patterns. Catalyzed by recent economic and social developments and facilitated by improved contraceptive technology, the phenomenon of childlessness is becoming increasingly acceptable to the public as the conflicts in traditional sex role and marriage patterns become more evident. Although the childless we have studied so far are predominantly from the middle class, recent survey data (Bram, 1978a) indicates that the trend towards childlessness is moving rapidly into the lower middle class and black populations. Childlessness as a lifestyle itself offers alternatives to traditional sex role definitions, but in addition facilitates a broad range of possibilities for diverging from sex role norms. We have seen this in the lifestyle and marriage patterns of the childless, as well as in their personal values and identities.

Childlessness also offers a critique of parenthood as it is currently organized in our society. The childless themselves speak of the way in which the burdens of parenthood fall so heavily on the isolated marital dyad, threatening the autonomy of the male and female and the closeness of the couple. Because of the current social expectations of mothers and sex role socialization, the burden falls more heavily on the female as men are prevented from participating as fully in the parental role. In order for men to share these activities more equitably, we would have to restructure the occupational system to include leave time and more flexible hours for both sexes, and guarantee economic security for women as well as men.

From our data we can extrapolate a fuller understanding of many of the contradictions we feel are intrinsic in current sex role definitions. For example, as parents, females are forced to choose between the traditionally neutralized sexuality of the mother in American society, and the erotic role of wife. The woman who has learned to defer to her husband or her employer in decision making, must develop her assertiveness and control once she is in charge of an infant, especially if she is then relegated to the homemaker role. The educated woman who has played the colleaguial, companionate role within marriage may find that the isolation of new motherhood is an interference with this role. Like a janus, the mother must focus inwards on the home and simultaneously outwards towards the "real" world.

Similar conflicts are instrinsic in the contemporary male role. For example, it is becoming increasingly clear that the modern woman chooses nurturant partners over Don Juans. Yet, men are still trained to demonstrate their masculinity through varying their sexual experiences. Similarly, the man who supports a family must move cautiously through the work world and make responsible decisions while exhibiting his courage and ability to take risks. These issues are clearly part of the male and female experience, with or without parenthood. The childless merely accentuate these difficulties in their refusal to accept one aspect of traditional sex role definitions.

NOTES

1 The following criteria were used to define the sample:
   Childless couples were aged a minimum of 21 years, married a minimum of one year, and, as determined in a preliminary interview, expressed the desire for no children, reported no physical fecundity impairment, and no history of previous children.
   Delay couples were of same age and marriage criteria, were currently childless but stated on preliminary interview that they intended to have children in the future.
   Parent couples were of same age and marriage criteria with their first child under the age of one year.
   Because of the small number and nonrandom distribution of the childless in the population the sample that was systematically chosen from the population of couples living in married students' housing had to be supplemented by subjects solicited through newspaper advertisements and informal referrals. An analysis of the groups by sample source yielded no significant differences, but there is still the possibility of self-selection affecting the results, as in all studies with volunteer subjects based on nonrandom samples.
2 In studying the motivations for childlessness, we utilized the fertility model based on the "values and costs" of children (Hoffman and Hoffman, 1973), developed to explain variations in fertility behavior, cultural differences and historical trends in the motivation to have children. The model is based on a framework of *values* that are tied to psychological needs and *costs*. The values are identified as:
   Adult status and social identity
   Expansion of the self, ties to a larger entity, immortality
   Morality: religion, altruism, good of the group
   Primary group ties, affiliation
   Stimulation, novelty, fun
   Creativity, accomplishment, competence
   Power, influence, effectance
   Social comparison, competition
   Economic utility

The costs were categorized in our study as:
Achievement
Structural (financial, time)
Marriage
Psychological (anxiety)
Dislike of children
Interference with spouse's life
Interference with lifestyle
World situation

3 Several studies have also investigated childlessness among lower middle class and lower class samples (Bram, 1978a, Nason & Poloma, 1976). Our own analysis of the national data collected by Hoffman (1975) indicates that the childless from a more representative sample than our original study are similar in most respects to the sample described here. One difference, however, is the extent to which the couples have developed an egalitarian marital style. The wives in this lower middle class sample are more likely to report that the husbands "help out" with household tasks rather than share them.

4 Rebecca (1977) followed up a portion of our original sample; the rest of the longitudinal follow-up is still in progress. She found that four years after the original interview the childless decision was still evolving and the reasons and attitudes toward childlessness, while basically the same, were in transition. For example, among the women, the reason most frequently given on re-interview was "lifestyle", as opposed to "achievement" concerns. The author attributes this to recent successes in achievement areas, as the subjects had finished school or obtained fulltime employment. The childless couples still placed great emphasis on the marriage and showed even less dissatisfaction with the amount of cohesiveness in the relationship than on the first interview, suggesting that the marital pattern had stabilized. The sex role orientations were evolving towards more egalitarianism.

5 Of the other studies on childlessness, two indicate that they did not find a statistically significant difference between the childless couples and comparison groups in their attitudes toward sex roles (Ory, 1978; Silka and Kiesler, 1977). However, in both cases the childless wives were more concerned with achievement goals than the others and could be interpreted as being less traditional in their sex role orientation.

REFERENCES

Blake, J.
1974 Can we believe recent data on birth expectations in the U.S.? Demography 11(1): 25–44.
Bram, S.
1974 To have or have not: A social psychological study of voluntarily childless couples, parents-to-be, and parents. Unpublished doctoral dissertation, University of Michigan, Ann Arbor, Michigan.
Bram, S.
1978 Through the looking glass: Voluntary childlessness as a mirror for contemporary changes in the meaning of parenthood. In W. R. Miller and L. F. Newman (eds.), The First Child and Family Formation. Chapel Hill, North Carolina: Carolina Population Center, pp. 368–391.
Bram, S.
1978a Update on childlessness. Paper presented at the meeting of the American Psychological Association, San Francisco, California.
den Bandt, M. L.
In progress. Project proposal on childlessness. Mimeographed.

Fawcett, J. T.
1973 Psychological Perspectives on Population. New York: Basic.
Gerson, M. J.
1977 Motivation for motherhood. Unpublished doctoral dissertation. New York University, New York.
Gustavus, S. O. and Henley, J. R.
1971 Correlates of voluntary childlessness in a select population. Social Biology 18: 277–284.
Hoffman, L. W. and Hoffman, M.
1973 The value of children to parents. In J. T. Fawcett (ed.), Psychological Perspectives on Population. New York: Basic, pp. 19–76.
Hoffman, L. W.
1974 Employment of women and fertility. In L. W. Hoffman, F. I. Nye (eds.), Working Mothers. San Francisco & London: Jossey-Bass, pp. 81–100.
Hoffman, L. W.
1975 The value of children to parents and the decrease in family size. Proceedings of the American Philosophical Society 119: 430–38.
Hoffman, L. W.
1977 Changes in family roles, socialization, and sex differences. American Psychologist 32(8): 644–657.
Houseknecht, S. K.
1977 Reference group support for voluntary childlessness: Evidence for conformity. Journal of Marriage and the Family 39(2): 285–293.
Nason, E. M. and Poloma, M. M.
1976 Voluntarily childless couples: The emergence of a variant lifestyle. Sage Research Papers in the Social Sciences. Series No. 90–040. Beverly Hills & London: Sage Publications.
Niphuis-Nell, M.
1976 Satisfactions and costs of children and fertility attitudes. Working papers of Netherlands Interuniversity Demographic Institute, No. 4.
Ory, M. G.
1978 The decision to parent or not: Normative and structural components. Journal of Marriage and the Family 40(3): 531–539.
Peck, E. and Senderowitz, J.
1974 Pronatalism: The Myth of Mom and Apple Pie. New York: Thomas Y. Crowell Company.
Pohlman, E.
1974 Changes in views towards childlessness: 1965–1970. In E. Peck, and J. Senderowitz, op. cit., pp. 276–277.
Rebecca, M.
1977 Stability and change in the lives of voluntarily childless couples. Unpublished doctoral dissertation. University of Michigan, Ann Arbor, Michigan.
Rozeboom, R.
1974 Motieven voor Vrijwillige Kinderloosheid. Groningen, Netherlands.
Silka, L. and Kiesler, S.
1977 Couples who choose to remain childless. Family Planning Perspectives 9(1): 16–25.
Thoen, G. A.
1977 Commitment among voluntary childfree couples to a variant lifestyle. Unpublished doctoral dissertation, University of Minnesota.
United States Bureau of the Census
1971 Current Population Reports, Series P-23, No. 36, 'Fertility indicators: 1970'.

United States Bureau of the Census
  1975 Current Population Reports, Series P–20, No. 279, 'Population profile of the United States: 1974'.
United States Bureau of the Census
  1976 Current Population Reports, Series P–20, No. 288, 'Fertility history and prospects of American women: June, 1975'.
Van Dusen, R. A., and Sheldon, E. B.
  1976 The changing status of American women: A life cycle perspective, American Psychologist: 106–116.
Veenhoven, R.
  1974 Is there an innate need for children? European Journal of Social Psychology 4(4): 495–501.
Veevers, J. E.
  1973 Voluntarily childless wives: An exploratory study. Sociology and Social Research 57: 356–366.
Veevers, J. E.
  1976 The life style of voluntarily childless couples. In L. Larsen (ed.), The Canadian Family in Comparative Perspective. Toronto: Prentice-Hall, pp. 394–411.
Whelan, E.
  1975 A Baby? . . . Maybe. New York: Bobbs-Merrill Company, Inc.
Westoff, C.
  1978 Some speculations on the future of marriage and fertility. Family Planning Perspectives 10: 79–83.

ADMA D'HEURLE, Ph.D.

CHANGING SEX ROLES REFLECTED IN THE FILMS OF FRANÇOIS TRUFFAUT

Serious scholarship relating to the meaning and aim of human sexuality and the changing definitions of sex roles has sought to place the question in a broad historical context. Since Kate Millet's evocative *Sexual Politics* a large number of studies have appeared dealing with the definition of femininity and masculinity at different periods in the history of western civilization and the relation of such definitions to the ethos of the epoch.[1] Beyond Margaret Mead's *Sex and Temperament*[2] anthropologists have also extended the inquiry horizontally to many cultures ranging from the very simple and traditional to the more complex and modern of western civilizations.

During the past year Michel Foucault has published the first volume of a multi-volume study of the history of human sexuality, a work which underscores the importance of a broad historical context for the contemporary search for a new understanding of the meaning of being man and women.[3] In this small volume Foucault draws a vivid sketch of the network of relations between the changing conceptions of sexuality and the styles of discourse, the economy of pleasure and the dynamics of power throughout the last three centuries. Foucault's insistence on this historical prespective gives new force to the message voiced by earlier works that without a dimension of depth the frantic contemporary search for the meaning of human sexuality and the most diligent efforts to decipher its language and its relations to pleasure, to utility, to power or to whatever the cultural tradition defines as the ultimate end of meaning of human existence are likely to be futile.

A comprehensive approach to the question of sex role definition is essential if the discourse is to go beyond the ascending crescendo of feminist politics. Susan Sontag's warning against the intellectual simplicity that is being demanded by feminist literature in the name of ethical solidarity must be taken seriously.[4]

It cannot be over-stressed that the intention of warnings against intellectual simplicity is not intended to muffle feminist criticism, to defuse the struggle against oppression or to discourage the search for clarification of the meanings we live by. To insist on the complexity of the issue at hand, is to call for humility and responsibility and point to the need for an intelligence that is not an instrument of authority, but an intelligence that is by Sontag's definition "critical, dialectical, skeptical and desimplifying".

With the broad scope of the problem in view, we have set ourselves the task of approaching the theme of attitudes towards sex roles through a study of love in the modern French film. A reflective look at the contemporary scene makes it quite evident that the movies are not simply another art form, a new recreational medium, an added element in an already encumbered social

I. Gross, J. Downing, and A. d'Heurle (eds.), Sex Role Attitudes and Cultural Change, 177–195.
Copyright © 1982 by D. Reidel Publishing Company.

environment. They are rather situations that bear a tremendous impact on feelings, motives, and behavior.

They are undeniably both important cultural artifacts and mirrors; looms for the weaving of individual dreams and cultural myths and a looking-glass reflecting images of those dreams and myths. The images of femininity and masculinity, of sex and love that are reflected in the modern film are an important source of enlightenment regarding the new sexuality and its meaning.

This study will focus on the work of Truffaut in which the theme of love and sex is prominent. The choice is based on the conviction that Truffaut is representative of a cinematic tradition, perhaps even a general aesthetic tradition where the interplay between the images of sex and romantic love has been a salient "existential motif". The claim that themes like love and sex tend to receive markedly different treatments in different cultural traditions finds support in the philosophy of aesthetics which has recognized the importance of a particular historical and linguistic matrix in which existential motifs are expressed. Ernst Cassirer's philosophy of symbolic forms, for example, puts emphasis on the forms of sensibility that are embodied in a special language and a particular cultural context.[5]

THE FRENCH VISION OF LOVE

A general familiarity with the French literary and aesthetic tradition reveals a sustained tension between the transcendental and the imminent, the eternal and the temporal, and the spiritual and the physical; a tension which also expresses itself in the saliency of the theme of interplay between romantic love and sex.

Studies of the modern film have often noted a difference in the treatment of the images of femininity and masculinity and the definitions of love and sex in the European versus the American film, but none, as far as we know, have gone beyond general descriptive statements or comments on particular films. In her authoritative study of the treatment of women in the movies, Molly Haskell discusses the genre of the woman's film as a particularly American phenomenon that is rooted in the circumscribed world of the American middle class woman as housewife, where "middle classness is not just an economic status but a state of mind and a relatively rigid moral code". Woman's film, which parented the later television soap opera, and depicted love as the "deadend of household drugery", Haskell sees as a particularly Anglo-Saxon phenomenon. In the European film she finds greater sensitivity to the role of women and subtlety in the treatment of the theme of love.[6] Stanley Kauffman in his reviews of modern French films has also noted the more nuanced treatment of the role of women and the absence of clear cut dichotomy between sex and love — marriage and romance.[7]

Examples can be multiplied to support the judgement of many a serious critic of the movies that the European film, particularly the film of the "new wave" in France has sustained a view of a complex but close relation between the physical sexual act and the experience of love. Strong support can be found for the hypothesis that this dialectic of sex and love has been an integral part of the French "Aesthetic world view" and that the modern French film in general and Truffaut's work in particular could be looked at as representatives of a tradition in which this particular "existential motif" has been played in different keys.

It will be remembered that it was the French historian Denis de Rougemont who did more than anyone else through his *Love in the Western World* to articulate the distinction between the tradition of romantic love which was born in the 12th century and the place of sex and marriage in society.[8] It is relevant to note, however, that when de Rougemont in a later work sought to demonstrate his thesis through the study of the novel, there was not one French novel in his sample.[9]

And Simone de Beauvior, who, in her classic *The Second Sex*,[10] takes the position that womanhood is defined through a cultural-historical process, also affirms a primary and immanent femininity. This affirmation stands out in her autobiography where she states that she never experienced the wish to be other than female and where she records with poignancy her struggle to win her freedom to be woman.[11] It is also present in her scholarly work where she takes great pains to demonstrate that there are no feminine values apart from masculine ones. This implied distinction between femininity and feminine roles is the first step towards qualifying a relationship between the sexes that could encompass both love and sexual desire. It is congruent with the ethos of the tradition of Denis de Rougemont, of Michael Foucault, of Stendhal of the "new wave" in film — a tradition that continues to reflect Dante's creed of love rather than that of the troubadours, the creed that does not separate human and divine love.

It is no accident that this tradition, which did not find a permanent and secure place for woman as goddess and which did not spiritualize love by separating it from desire, today produces a most unusual work that unabashedly revives the idiom of romantic love and speaks the language of tenderness and romantic folly and has come to ring more "obscene" than the language of the body. It comes from France — and unusual work by Roland Barthes[12] to reaffirm what Jean Guitton years ago called the manifest difference between "problem" and "mystery":

A problem is a difficulty caused by ignorance; it can, therefore, be resolved by knowledge. A mystery is a difficulty concerning nature or a thing in itself which knowledge increases. If society makes a problem of sex it is because of its impotence to dissipate the mystery.

The special meaning, for our time, of Truffaut's image of human sexuality lies in its faithfulness to a tradition that has grappled with the problem without dissipating the mystery.

TRUFFAUT AND THE ART OF THE CINEMA

As we seek to locate Truffaut in the world of film we find him among the fathers of the "new wave", a group of French cinema artists who in the early nineteen fifties forged a new film theory. The two focal points of the new collective theory were the questions of film genres and the "politique des auteurs", a phrase attributed to Truffaut himself. The new film theory gave explicit recognition to the importance of the interaction between the history of the art and the evaluation of the artist's personal style. Hence a full appreciation of Truffaut's vision requires an understanding of the "deep structure" of his *oeuvres* in terms of his central themes and the style in which they are cast (lyrical, ironic, nostalgic, etc.) as well as his use of particular cinematic genres such as crime melodrama, romance, comedy slapstick, etc.

In regard to themes, all of the films that Truffaut has made, about two score to date, are essentially explorations in the meaning of love and art. He has experimented with a variety of genres but in all of them the same fundamental themes resonate in a lyrical, low-keyed, disciplined style that brings together effortlessly the comic and the tragic and does it with a most effective and distinctive sense of irony. Our interest here is particularly in his treatment of love and every film that Truffaut has made is essentially about love. Central, of course, is the love of man and woman, but there is also the generational love of adults and children and the human, communal setting that is required to sustain them. These forms of love, the sexual and the generational, are closely related to one another and each is intertwined with the meaning of language and of work.

GENERATIONAL LOVE

Only three of Truffaut's twenty or so films deal primarily with generational love: *The Four Hundred Blows* (1959), *The Wild Child* (1969), and *Small Change* (1976). However, the theme of parental nurturance appears in many of the other films. In the three major films dealing with adult and child, the relation of language and work to the experience of nurturance is most subtly and effectively underscored.

In the world of Antoine in *The Four Hundred Blows* work has no meaning, whether it be the work of his parents which the city conceals, that of his teachers which barley touches his life, or the work of the psychologist whose questioning embodies the voice of incomprehension. Language in its written form is important for Antoine. His youthful adoration of Balzac is significant and his admiration of *Quest for the Absolute* establishes a relationship between the written word, art, literature, and the ideal which is one of Truffaut's most persistent themes. The world of the written word and the realm of the absolute, however, have no connection either with the spoken word or with Antoine's existential reality. Conversation with adults has so little meaning for him that we are not in the least surprised by his answer to the psychologist regarding his lying; "Well, I lie sometimes, but so what? When I tell them the truth they don't believe me anyway".

From the world of Antoine who "missed being loved, who grows up without tenderness"[14] Truffaut moved in *The Wild Child* to a world where the learning and teaching of language becomes the focus of a human community where love and work are one. The most recent of the three films dealing with generational love, *Small Change* uses the same elements but in addition ties together the love of the child with the sexual love of man and woman. It is perhaps this fruitful harmony, towards which Truffaut's compassionate imagination has been moving since he took camera in hand, that illuminates the film and gives it a special verve.

THE AUTOBIOGRAPHICAL FILMS

The images of sexual love in Truffaut are most clearly reflected in the auto-biographical works which depict most directly *l'education sentimentale* of Antoine Doinel, the Truffaut surrogate. These films fall, according to the most widely accepted chronological ordering of his work, in the first period which covers his film-making career roughly until 1964, and the third period, which began in 1968. The first is a short little-known work entitled *Les Mistons* (1958), which prefaces in subject matter and style the four major works in the series: *The Four Hundred Blows, Love at Twenty, Stolen Kisses* and *Bed and Board.*

The Four Hundred Blows continues the theme of awakening sexuality and introduces through the portrait of thirteen-year-old Antoine, the Truffaut hero with the sensitive, innocent, vulnerable and diffident manner, struggling to come to terms with woman and with love.

Love at Twenty (1962) and *Stolen Kisses* (1968) develop this portrait further as they pursue Antoine's quest. At the beginning of the first of the two Antoine is sixteen, independent and newly launched into the world of work. The film establishes this quickly with opening shots of his living quarters and the record publishing company where he works. The intoxicating love-at-a-distance which sweeps him off his feet follows inevitably. There are numerous exchanges of records and letters. Antoine offers Colette the first record that he makes, which she accepts with the same indifference with which she receives his caresses. The film ends with Antoine rejected by his beloved but accepted by her family.

In *Stolen Kisses* the polarization of the images of women and the dichotomy between romantic love and lust are depicted more sharply. Here Antoine's search to establish his adult masculine identity is more focused. It is in essence a search to know who he is in relation to the women in his life. The sexual prowess and sophistication that the young Antoine tries to assume upon his visits to the prostitutes in the first part of the film only highlight his innocence and his fear of women. He first appears in this film in the military barracks prison reading Balzac's story of unconsummated love, *The Lily of the Valley.*

On the way to the officer who will announce to him his dishonorable discharge, he hears the adjutant in the barrack classroom making the comparison between the dangerous business of dismantling mines and "handling women".

Out of the army, he is again alone at the edge of conventional society an outsider in search of work and of love. The visit to his old girlfriend Christine's home is reminiscent of his relation with Colette's parents in *Love at Twenty*. With Christine herself, things do not go smoothly; she is too matter of fact to fit his romantic dream of the unattainable goddess, and the sexual advances used in casual relations with prostitutes do not impress her. But a goddess soon appears in the shape of Fabienne Tobard, the beautiful wife of the shoe store owner where Antoine's work as a private detective had brought him. Regarding Fabienne as an embodiment of the absolute love that in the Truffaut film so far is totally divested from the real everyday existence, Don Allen writes:

Fabienne Tabard, dream goddess and fairytale princess, is Antoine's Damascus road vision, inspiring in him awed veneration and complete enslavement. This image of beatified purity and mystic inner radiance is made for worship.[15]

Antoine's report to the detective agency endorses his romantic vision and underscores the absurdity of both his idolatry and his work.[16] Antoine's yearning for the perfect love is beautifully portrayed against shots of the Sacré Coeur suggesting a wider dimension to Antoine's infatuation and his yearning for the ideal. His farewell letter to his "lady" is a modern troubadour song. The answer is no apparition but Fabienne herself. With candor, sensitivity and intelligence she breaks through his romantic dream. Fabienne does not mock Antonine's sentiments nor does she dismiss his reference to Balzac. She simply asserts:

I am not an apparition, I am a woman . . . You say that I am exceptional. That's true, I am exceptional. But then, every woman is exceptional . . . each in her own way. You over there, you are certainly exceptional . . . you are unique. We are, each of us unique . . . unique and irreplaceable.[17]

Fabienne has brought Antoine a long way on his journey towards a new vision of love and a new knowledge of himself. The moving and humorous scene of Antoine in front of the mirror repeating his name and the names of the two women in his life are of the past. Not that the delicate tension between the face and the mask, the ideal and the provisional, the illusion and the reality is fully dissipated. The "deep structure" of the Truffaut film belies the possibility that this tension could be totally removed. This moment in the life of the hero simply marks the critical period in his psychosexual development where he comes to apprehend that life must encompass both realms; that the love he seeks must be the love of a real woman as well as an abstract ideal.

Antoine leaves Fabienne less terrified of the actuality of love and more confirmed in his intuitive apprehension that sexual love is an assertion of life in the face of death. After the climatic encounter with Fabienne, Antoine is ready to go back to Christine and the rest of the film conveys a buoyant spirit of promise for the new love.

The breakfast scene after Antoine and Christine had spent the night together is charged with symbols of hope. Antoine puts the coils of a bottle opener around Christine's ring finger as they look into each others' eyes and smile. The proposed marriage will not be a conventional affair as the bottle opener indicates, neither will it be devoid of romance as is indicated by the mysterious written messages that are exchanged. It will also aspire to mutuality as Christine and Antoine promise to teach each other all they know. In the final scene in the park Antoine and Christine are approached by the stranger who has been following Christine for days, and who now awkwardly makes his declaration of love, ending with the grandiose finale, "For I am definitive". Christine dismisses the incident with a shrug of the shoulder, but Antoine is visibly disturbed. His expression saves the film from putting closure on its statement regarding the two-dimensional natural of love.

Bed and Board brings a new dimension to Antoine's quest and Truffaut's explorations into the meaning of love by taking into account the woman's perspective. The conjugal setting in itself does not necessitate this extension for one can easily consider the continuation of Antoine's story uniquely from his point of view. The films could have been made with a wife cast in a strictly conventional role, but Truffaut chooses to shift the focus to include both man and woman. Christine is not portrayed as a stereotyped middle class wife. She is a competent violinist, an artist herself. She is not, like many earlier Truffaut female characters, the artistic creation of a man.

Consistency with the thrust of *Stolen Kisses* requires the development of a new dialectic of love. Fabienne's message, "woman is exceptional . . . each of us is unique . . . unique and irreplaceable", necessitates the development of Antoine's partner in love as a three-dimensional being. Not only the man, but woman too must come to terms with her sexuality if the couple is going to survive and come to terms with paternity. The task requires meaningful communication between lovers and significant relations between the couple and the larger community. The persistent presence of the courtyard as if it were itself a character in this film symbolizes the broader social context against which the microcosm of the couple is sustained.

The discomfort that Antoine and Christine experience in their sexual relations is expressed in various ways throughout the first part of the film (reaction to nudity, the humorous exchange about Christine's breasts, etc.). It is most pointedly indicated in the Abelard and Isolde scene where they are together in bed each reading a book about the opposite sex. However, their openness and candor with one another, the sense of humor they share, and their obvious pleasure in one another compensate for the dis-ease and provide the antidote for Antoine's short-lived romantic obsession with Kyoko.

The spell of the new goddess of love is explained by her being an exotic Japanese woman who stands outside the hubbub of everyday life; outside the world of necessity and of work; "a different continent". The character of Kyoko gives the film-maker an excellent opportunity to highlight the importance of language which is so fundamental to his theory of love. Throughout Truffaut's work written language is associated with the absolute, and the spoken word with the provisional and the real. In the realm of love, the romantic yearning for the unattainable *l'amour fou* is always expressed in letters and written messages. But love in the real world according to *Stolen Kisses* and *Bed and Board* requires conversation because it takes into account the reality of the beloved. Antoine's romantic attachment to Kyoko is maintained for a brief period by ritualistic and stylized modes of communication appropriate for worship. Boredom drives Antoine repeatedly to the telephone to speak with Christine, and eventually back to live with her, "the woman with whom he is never bored". At another level Kyoko's declaration that Antoine is the man with whom she would most like to commit suicide suggests, even through its humorous irony, an assoiacation of death with ideal love and a new affirmation that shared sexual love is an assertion of life in the face of death.

At the end of *Bed and Board* Antoine emerges, not as the idealized glamorous "Romantic Hero", but a more modern "anti-hero" embroiled in the messiness of everyday life. He has left Kyoko, he is almost finished writing his novel, and he has returned to Christine who is not satisfied to be his sister, daughter and mother but wants to be also his wife. At the end of the film, Christine herself is better prepared to be a wife for Antoine. This is suggested by her recognition of her own initial fear of sex and her assertion that despite everything Anotine had done, she still loves him and is never bored with him. But even more persuasively her growth is revealed in her autonomy and her sense of personal responsibility which express themselves in her actions as well as her words.

The autobiographical films of Truffaut give the theme of love its most direct and accessible expression. However, to limit the exploration of the theme to these films is to do a grave injustice to Truffaut as a artist and to his theory of film which insists on the importance of the cinema's "language" as well as its "style"; its "genres" as well as its *auteurs*. A comprehensive analysis of the nature of love and its relation to language and to work should ideally include all the films that he has made particularly since he himself has often stressed the central position that the theme occupies in all his work. Limitations on the scope of this paper, however, makes a detailed analysis of the variations on the theme of love in all of Truffaut's films impossible. An attempt will be made to consider the films where these variations are more resonant.

LITERARY AND PSYCHOLOGICAL FILMS – THE EARLY PERIOD

The autobiographical films through which we have attempted to trace a change in Truffaut's vision of love, span a long period of time, from 1958 to 1970. It would be of value to determine whether a similar change is discernible in his other major films over this same period of time and beyond it to the present. The task takes us most naturally back to *Shoot the Piano Player*, one of Truffaut's earliest works. This film followed *The Four Hundred Blows* and puzzled the admirers who expected another in the same idiom. It also dazzled the critics with its stylistic virtuosity and bold departures from traditional modes. This film, which has come to be considered a classic in the history of the cinema, is of particular interest from the point of view of this study, primarily for its preoccupation with love, its explicit association of romantic love with death and its faint suggestion of the possibility of real love. The hero, Charlie/Edouard, is the embodiment of the romantic ideal for two women, Therese and Lena, who are sacrificed for him. The love and lust dilemma is involved in Therese's sacrifice of herself for the sake of Charlie's career as a concert pianist. Her suicide follows a confession which breaks a long, anguished silence, and could have been avoided had Charlie found his words of reassurance in time.

One of the most memorable features of this film is the character of its hero, Charlie Kohler. The identity of the winning hero is complex; he is a recluse who is drawn into the midst of the action; a self-proclaimed puritan who has sexual relations with three women; a passive pawn in the fact of chance who chooses a new life for himself; a gentle man who commits murder; an expert concert pianist who pounds on a piano in a bistro. The contradictions can be multiplied. This complicated man whose fractured image gives a degree of unity to the disordered universe of the film, has many of the qualities of the typical Truffaut hero.[18] One of the most most subtly expressed qualities which gains prominence in the character of the heroes of the later films is that elusive quality of being a man capable of loving and being loved by woman.

Shoot the Piano Player was followed by *Jules and Jim* (1961), which remains to this day one of Truffaut's most popular films. It was one of the last films of Truffaut's first period.

This period was followed by six years of experimentation with various film genres, ending with the return in 1968 to the autobiographical Antonine Doinel series. *The Soft Skin* (1964), *Fahrenheit 451* (1966), and *The Bride Wore Black* (1968) belong to this period. Although these films are of interest primarily as experiments in genre they definitely have the trademark of their author. Truffaut himself spoke of the freedom that the genre film gave him by distancing him from his subject matter. Speaking particularly of *Stolen Kisses* he said, "I had to constantly cover my tracks, camouflage myself, and transpose so that I wouldn's be too recognizable. In short, I wore a mask. In *The Bride Wore Black* . . . on the contrary, the mask existed 'a priori', and behind borrowed characters, I felt freer to express my own personality".[19]

The above three genre films, their fixed structure notwithstanding, tell a great deal about Truffaut's vision of love. They convey his preoccupation with relation and isolation, his association of the written word with *l'amour fou*, and the further association of this form of oneway passion with obsession and with death. Although a closer analysis of the three films of Truffaut's experimental period would indeed be fruitful, we must restrict our comments to this brief mention of them and turn to the literacy and psychological films where the treatment of the theme of love is necessarily less masked. *Jules and*

Jim and *Two English Girls* will be considered together inspite of the long decade that separates them. Both films are based on novels by Henri-Pierre Roche and have many stylistic and thematic similarities; one film being the story of two men in love with one woman and the other of two women in love with one man. *Jules and Jim* begins with a portrait of the friendship of two young men in pre-war Paris. The friends are different in many ways; Jules is German, small and blond, systematic and persistent in his approach to things, and has limited experience with women; Jim is French, tall and dark, casual in his comportment, curious and wide-ranging in his interests. Unlike Jules he has numerous relationships with women. The two men enjoy a deep affection for one another and have many common interests. They are both writers and share a love for language and literature.

A slide of a woman's face on a statue , shown them by an acquaintance, captivates both of them. They decide to go to an island in the Adriatic to see the original and there:

They stayed by the statue for an hour. It exceeded all their expectations, and they walked and walked rapidly round and round it, without saying a word . . . Not until the following day did they talk about it . . . Had they ever met that smile before? Never ! . . . What would they do if they met it one day? They would follow it.[20]

Soon after, Catherine, whose face bore a strange resemblance to the statue comes into their life. In the same way that *Shoot the Piano Player* centers on Charlie, *Jules and Jim* focuses on Catherine. Her connection with the statue establishes her immediately as an archetypal figure, an "incarnation of the life force", a goddess whom the two men will worship and by whom they will ultimately be destroyed.

During the first half of the film, Catherine appears as a blithe spirit who lives in the moment and, like the character in the play within the film, "she wants to be free. She invents her life every moment".[21] The freedom is deceptive, for Catherine is imprisoned by what Monaco calls "the burden of symbolhood".[22] From the moment that the eyes of the two men fall on her she becomes a projection of their fantasies. Any chance that she may have been understood as a person was removed when the rendez-vous with Jim at the cafe was missed. Waiting for her, Jim for the first time found himself thinking of her as a person. But Catherine did not appear and the possibility that she would have come into existence as a real woman did not materialize.

This climactic episode is reinforced by the arrival of the war. "The revolting thing about war", said Jules, "is that it deprives a man of his own individual struggle".[23] The existential struggle is suspended. Images are frozen and communication becomes limited to letters. Catherine marries Jules after the war. Later she explains to Jim:

He wrote me marvellous, passionate love-letters. I loved him more at a distance. Once again I saw him with a halo. Our final misunderstanding, the real rupture, came on his first leave. I felt I was in the arms of a stranger.[24]

Catherine's imprisonment in her role as idol, and her own total identification with this person explain her need to be at the center of attention at all times. It also explains her obsession with winning and her disregard for rules. Life for her is a performance, a kind of game for which she whimsically devises her own rules.

Paradoxically, the imprisonment provides freedom from conventional roles as well as from accepted moral and ethical codes. It also provides Catherine with the possibility of expressing masculine aspects of her personality as when she appears disguised as a man. C. G. Crisp points to this androgynous quality as a major source of her magic.[25]

Catherine's freedom from conventional regulations and established ethical codes, the freedom to actualize her androgyny could have been a positive force. Instead, it brough only destruction into her world because it was the freedom of an abritrary power that "expressed itself in cataclysms", that knew no responsibility, no justice, no past and no future. At the end of the film, Jim comes to see this and attempts to share his knowledge with Catherine, but it is then too late.

In as much as the film has centered on Catherine, critical comment has tended to stress its fairytale character and ignore the psychological dynamics of the relationships among the triad. It is, therefore, important to stress the fact that the film itself underscores these relationships. Catherine is the goddess that Jules and Jim identify with the statue and its permanence, but she is also the woman who is maintained as their creation, the projection of their fantasies. Catherine comes into their life as a goddess and remains, even in marriage, a stranger. Jules' possessive constancy isolates her from her existential struggle, as the war deprives him of his. This constancy on Jules' part is paralleled by Jim's rejection of marriage and his insistence on an equally deceptive freedom in his relation to Gilberte.

The film makes it clear that neither Jules' constancy, nor Jim's rejection of responsibility allow for the existential struggle that love requires if it is to survive. While it is true that Jules and Gilberte, the two faithful members of each couple survive, the film is far from being a hymn to constancy. It is ironic that the sympathies of the audience are bent towards the faithful lovers, particularly Jules, because the film emphasizes the relation of the absolutism in love, which cuts out the world, to the death that ends the film. The answer to the dilemma posed by *Jules and Jim* lies in its affirmation of the need for the "individual's own struggle", which implies a search for meaningful freedom and responsibility in love.

FILMS OF THE LATER PERIOD

The similarities between *Two English Girls* and *Jules and Jim* are many. Stylistically there is similarity in the sweeping views of magnificently romantic landscapes and in the use of the contrast between outdoor and indoor and country and city scenes: the metaphoric use of trains, windows and stairs; the means of marking the passage of time, etc.

In the treatment of the same theme of love in its permanent-temporary, romantic-real, spiritual-physical aspects, however, we find notable differences underlying the obvious commonality. *Two English Girls* is a far more explicitly psychological film. Its focus on the triangular relationship is more intense and the emotional obstacles that keep the characters apart are less obscure. This film was produced immediately after *Bed and Board* where we found Truffaut to be more sensitive to the perspective of a woman in love. In his treatment of Anne and Muriel, the two English girls, he extends and gives a much fuller account of the complex struggle involved in the surrender of the ideal of purity in love. The two sisters are set in the puritanical atmosphere of rural England at the turn of the century but the fears, the inhibitions and the self-deceptions that stand between the characters and their actions are by no means the simple outcome of a Victorian morality.

Anne is an artist, a sculptress curious to explore the world and to participate in its creation, and Muriel is an introvert, an absolutist, a diarist who needs to be in control of her world. She has sensitive eyes and wears a bandage to protect them.

Claude's written declaration of love to Muriel does not bring an end to the self-deceptions but precipitates the forced separation. Back in Paris, Claude enjoys the world of art and casual sexual relations and writes to Muriel indicating his desire to renounce marriage. Sometime later he discovers Anne and the two have an affair which will not be Anne's only one. Muriel sends her diary to Claude, who finds in her intimate confessions of erotic desire "material for a novel". She herself arrives in Paris and Claude finds himself again between the two sisters. Muriel's advances are disturbing to him and he is incapable of approaching her. For him Muriel has remained a goddess of "terrifying purity". Muriel's response to the truth about the relation between Claude and Anne is a violent physical reaction. After Anne's death of tuberculosis Muriel and Claude meet in Calais and their sexual encounter is unique in Truffaut for its violently passionate quality.

In contrast with the gentle tenderness of his love encounter with Anne, here all is brutal passion as Claude unintentionally 'provides Muriel with a weapon to use against him' . . . and blood fills the screen. The rupture of Muriel's chastity is symbolic of the rupture of the ties that have bound her to Claude for seven years . . . [26]

The amorous goddess, although not a "different continent", is from a different land. "I come to bury us" she explains to her lover and after her conquest, leaves him to return to England to marry and bear a child. The trains crossing each other at the station going in different directions symbolize the painful and final separation of the lovers. Muriel will not stay with Claude although she admits that she can live without him as she can live without eyes or legs. Claude is left in Paris to write his memories and the story of his love for the two foreign sisters.

In *Two English Girls*, the demand of the ideal does not lead to death as it does in *Jules and Jim*, and *Shoot the Piano Player*, both films of an earlier period. Having come together in burning passion Muriel and Claude separate, one to live within conventional marriage and the other to eternalize the memory of their love in a book. The film's ending is a poignant reminder that the myth of the separation between Eros and Agape, which Denis de Rougemont traces back to the twelfth century, is still alive. The power of the film lies not in its invocation of the myth but in the question mark that it ends with. Its open-endedness leaves the audience with the unresolved tension between the love that requires distance, and that which seeks the reality of the other; between the mystery of the myth and the compelling problem of the individual lovers.

Truffaut said that he wanted *Two English Girls* to be a physical film on love, rather than a film on physical love. This he accomplished through the vivid portrayal of the violence of Muriel and Claude's sexual passion as well as the repeated images of blood and tears and vomit. The imagery of the film leaves no doubt that love is not worship of an idol; it is not even affection based on mutual respect and liking, but it is a physical force, a torrent in the river of life.

Nowhere else in Truffaut's films do we find as strong a statement regarding the role of sexuality and the need for love to come to terms with it. In this film he comes closer than ever before to an understanding of love as *sentiment*, in the full meaning of the French word. For it is true that *sentiment* is charged with more intellectual connotations than the English word 'feeling', but it is equally true that it keeps at its very root the presence of *sens* in its concrete and bodily meaning.

In the context of Truffaut's work, the sexual encounter between Muriel and Claude has especial significance. It is certainly not a concession to popular sensationalism or the current trend to link sex with violence. The meaning of this love scene, which has puzzled many a Truffaut admirer, can be understood only as another statement about the nature of love by an artist whose work has been devoted to its study.

The note of optimism that was struck in *Stolen Kisses* is sustained by *Bed and Board* which brings back together within marriage the couple that can talk together, share what they know and are "never bored with one another". The promise of *Bed and Board* must not be mistaken for Truffaut's final answer, congruent as it might be with an enlightened, modern and widely accepted view of love. The view, common among today's young adult generation, that love is no more than mutual liking and a sharing of ideas and ideals is not endorsed by Truffaut. Mutuality is important. It is necessary as *Stolen Kisses* and *Bed and Board* indicate but it is not enough. The other films of this period bring into focus the reality of sex and the mystery of the other. They also envision a process of development through which such rich and complex love comes into being.

THE LATER WORKS

It is perhaps Truffaut's insistence on love as a process that can be actualized through existential strife that has led many a student of modern film to describe his vision as basically pessimistic. Close study of the films of Truffaut's third period, on the contrary, reveals an optimistic outlook regarding the love of man and woman.

After years of research in the myths of love in the Western World Denis de Rougemont asks:

If it is true that the Other as such remains the best defended mystery in the eyes of a demanding love – could Eros and Agape not join in a paradoxical alliance at the very heart of accepted marriage?[27]

The later films of Truffaut suggest a positive answer to de Rougemont's question. The alliance of Eros and Agape is possible if the love of man and woman can incorporate the reality as well as the mystery of the Other. After *Stolen Kisses* the faith in the possibility of this alliance appears more firm. *Mississippi Mermaid* produced in the same year reflects this faith. It is the story of the love an idealist, Louis Mahe, a bachelor of thirty-seven who decides to end his loneliness by advertising for a wife in the personal columns of a newspaper. The ideal woman of his dreams materializes in the person of a woman of dubious character who robs him of his money and attempts to escape. The major part of the film is an account of the struggle of Louis and Marion, the new goddess of death, beyond the law at the fringe of society. Truffaut avoids the expected tragic ending of the melodrama (and the novel's ending for that matter). Louis' real love for Marion makes it impossible for him to kill her, as he had intended. His devotion through-out their struggle to escape from the authorities is constant and survives the harsh realities of poverty and danger. Ultimately it moves Marion.

Death in *Mississippi Mermaid* does not result from the abandonment of the ideal. The couple survive and the last image of them walking through the snow towards the Swiss border ends the film with the promise that the love of a man who described himself as belonging to a "race of idealists that try to find defini-tive happiness in seven lines of a newspaper advertisement", can endure as it is transformed and shared. The romantic ideal and sensual sexuality become associated with violence and death only when they are separated from love as an *élan* towards the reality as well as the mystery of the Other.

In *Adele H.* (1967), Truffaut returns to the filming of romantic love from yet another perspective. Adele's love remains a solitary adventure and her passion becomes an obsession that costs her sanity and seals her soul from the world of reality. This severance was symbolized by the hand on the beloved's lips to prevent him from speaking at their first meeting after Adele had crossed the ocean in search for him. There is irony in her soliloquy,

I can learn everything by myself; but for love, I need him. When we meet, I will tell him: "If one of us doesn't love enough to want marriage above all else, then it isn't love."[28]

Adele's need excludes Pinson's reality and her love of him seeks only the "lyrical impulse of its narration".

Before Adele leaves the relative security of the Saunders' home where she had been watched over, to begin her rapid decline towards destitution, another image is superimposed on the present. It is the image of a young girl standing by the sea facing the waves as if she herself were on the water, with a hopeful faraway look in her eyes. Adele's young voice is heard saying: "This incredible thing – that a young girl shall walk over the sea, from the Old into the New World, to join her lover – this, I shall accomplish".[29] The same image is repeated at the end of the film with the narrator reciting the same words that Adele had written in her diary fifty years earlier.

The miracle can be understood in many ways, of course, particularly as Truffaut uses the water image in relation to nightmares which evoke the drowning of the sister and her young husband, and as a background to Adele's letter that travels over the ocean telling her parents lies about her prospective marriage. The miracle of Adele's love may be in part fantasy and in part deception. It is still nevertheless a miracle manifest in the survival of the story of that love through Adele's memoirs and Truffaut's recreation of the story in beautiful images. Furthermore, the miracle lies in the power of the story of Adele's love, that has survived for over a century, to move, so powerfully, the modern imagination.

Small Change (1976) is the last film of Truffaut to be shown so far outside of France.[30] It is a delightful film about children which appears deceptively simple because of its playful, low-keyed and very personal style. Close examination of this recent film in the light of the whole body of Truffaut's work show it to be of particular significance in revealing the multi-dimensional image of love that Truffaut has examined from so many different perspectives. What Collin Westerback said in his review of *Adele H.* remains ever so true one film later,

The further along Truffaut's career progresses, the harder it is to respond to any new film by itself. Each work is so richly entangled with all the films that have preceded it, it seems Truffaut's whole career must be reviewed with each new film that appears.[31]

Looking at *Small Change* as an extension of Truffaut's explorations in the nature of love, the film becomes a harmonious mosaic in which the many points and counterpoints that the previous films have made about love fall in place. The film begins in front of a landmark at the "exact center of France" with twelve year-old Martine mailing a post card to her cousin. The post card from Bruere-Allichamps, contemplated by cousin Raoul, becomes the subject of discussion in Jean-François Richet's class. The address is written on the blackboard, explanation is given and personal comment is invited. The class scene quickly establishes M. Richet as a man who loves children and his work with them. This love, which individualizes the children, cannot be separated from his love for his pregnant wife Lydie. The sexual love of the couple is placed in the context of the wider community. It is an intergal aspect of the freedom it gives the couple to relate to other adults as persons, and to children with honesty and candor.

Communication both written and oral and its relation to the love between man and woman, and between adults and children is the underlying theme of *Small Change*. The opening scene sets the tone for the type of communication that Jean-François Richet has with the children in his class. There is the same warmth and honesty in his conversations with his colleague Chantal Petit. Lydie, his wife, talks with her neighbors, adults and children with the same openness. The conjugal life of the couple is at the heart of the film and it informs their relation with the community. The miracle of their love is by no means attenuated by the domestic realities which are emphasized by the disorder necessitated by their move to a new apartment, and is rekindled by the wondrous birth of their child:

In the hospital's delivery room M. Richet stands holding his father's old rolleiflex, ready to take pictures of the birth of the child ... Jean-François suddenly looks like a little boy again, and his wide-eyed expression is very similar to Richard's.[32]

Jean-François, the loving husband and beloved teacher, is also the artist with the child-like faculty for awe and wonder.

In the children's discussion of the birth there are insinuations of a relationship between sexuality and impurity. The unsavory tone is dissipated when the teacher arrives and puts an end to the children's speculations. He answers their questions candidly and writes the baby's name on the blackboard. The assurance makes it possible to extend the the connection back to sex comfortably and one of the children is able to ask, "And how is your wife?" Jean-François also answers this question with a big smile. The trust revealed in this conversation between the adult and the children soon extends to action when the children are asked to forfeit the toy guns that had been illegally acquired.

The perennial Truffaut theme of written language and oral dialogue resonates in the brief nursing scene. Lydie is breast-feeding the baby, and the young father stops while arranging his books on a shelf to read to her from a book by Bettelheim,

While breast-feeding, the infant is well aware whether he is being held in an anxious or a relaxed manner ... The infant's well-being or unease will influence his entire future behavior, and his later relationships with women will depend directly on his initial relationship with his mother.[33]

The intellectual simplicity, if not triteness, of this scene is averted through the humorous irony with which Lydie responds to the "lesson". In her manner and in her answer there is reassurance about the quality of their own relationship. There is also a deeper irony about the determinism reflected in the statement that was read. Later in the film Jean-François is talking with the children about Julien, who had been removed from his home where he had been cruelly treated. He tells them,

It is because I have bitter memories of my own childhood and because I don't like the way children are being treated that I have chosen this profession, that I've chosen to be a teacher.

Life is not easy, it is hard, and it is important that you steel yourselves in order to meet it. I am not telling you to become callous, I am telling you to grow strong.[34]

Underly his admonishing is the assumption that man enjoys a margin of freedom and support for the final statement of the film that the children are impatient to "lead their lives".

The film in its complex mosaic incorporates many sub-plots; the most important perhaps from the perspective of this study is the story of Patrick Desmouceaux. Patrick lives with, and takes care of, a crippled father. In his care for his kind father Patrick shows unusual responsibility. His infatuation with the mother of one of his friends is reminiscent of *Les Mistons* and the young Antoine Doinel. At the end of the film Patrick is at summer camp, in love with Martine, the girl whose card from the center of France opened the film. Martine writes about their love, their first kiss and the uproar when they got back to the refectory. The film ends with the narrator's description of the uproar,

It is not a hostile noise, nor is it particularly friendly; it is just a great noise, an explosion of vital energy. All the shouts and yells and laughter light up a hundred and twenty children's faces, sixty boys and sixty girls, and those faces all similar, all different, remind one of a Chinese crowd: They are the faces of children who are impatient to lead their lives.[35]

The cyclic pattern introduced through the story of Patrick and Martine's awakening sexuality, is not new in Truffaut. In the early films, particularly *Shoot the Piano Player* and *Jules and Jim*, when continuity and repetition are suggested, they are the mechanical continuity and repetitiveness of obsession and death, of the blind wheels of destiny grinding on. Truffaut's return to the theme of pre-adolescent love is not an automatic repetition. In regard to his filming the same situation he writes,

By now, I am obviously aware that I have a predilection for films of sentiment . . . Within each picture, I run into the conflict between temporary, and definitive sentiments, so that *I seem to be filming the same situations.*

Those who have affinity for these subjects — the lowkey description of strong emotion — will see them as variants on a theme. Those who are bored with them will say that I repeat myself.[36]

The love of Patrick and Martine is a variation on a theme. The romantic love of youth is here cast in a new light. After the many films that intervened between *Les Mistons* and *Small Change*, it becomes evident that the new-born love of the young couple need not of necessity be bound to illusion, separateness and death. Patrick is a dreamer whose feet are firmly grounded in reality. He is bound to the older generation as much through his love and responsible care for his father as through his infatuation with his friend's mother. And Martine

194ADMA D'HEURLE

welcomes their first kiss as she insists on recording in written words the beauty of the miracle of their new love. At the closing of the film Patrick and Martine are seen among the other children, "Anxious to lead their lives" and to under-take their "individual struggle". The freedom available to them may allow the nurturance of the sentiment which has been born to develop into a rich love capable of coming to terms with the fullness of being of the Other. The couple at the center of the film offer a testimony that such love is possible. Jean-François Richet who is the embodiment of the romantic hero of previous films, is a man who can love woman with a love that maintains its awe of the miraculous, speaks its name and translates it into meaningful relatedness to the world.

Mercy College, Dobbs Ferry, New York

NOTES

1   Miller, Kate, Sexual Politics (New York: Avon, 1971).
2   Mead, Margaret, Sex and Temperament in Three Primitive Societies (New York: William Morrow, 1935).
3   Foucault, Michel, La Volonté de Savoir (Paris: Gallimard, 1976).
4   Sontag, Susan, 'Notes on Art, Sex and Politics,' New York Times, 8 February 1976, sec. 2, p. 36.
5   Cassirer, Ernst, Language and Myths (New York: Dover Publishing Co., 1946).
6   Haskell, Molly, From Reverence to Rape (Baltimore: Penguin Books, 1974), pp. 284–285.
7   Kauffman, Stanley, 'Chloë in the Afternoon', The New Republic, 14 October 1972, p. 22.
8   de Rougemont, Denis, Love in the Western World (New York: Pantheon, 1956).
9   de Rougemont, Denis, Love Declared (New York: Pantheon, 1963).
10 de Beauvoir, Simone, The Second Sex (New York: Knopf, 1953).
11 de Beauvoir, Simone, Memoirs of a Dutiful Daughter (New York: World 1959), p. 55.
12 Barthes, Roland, Fragments d'un Discours Amoureux (Paris: Éditions du Seuil, 1977).
13 Guitton, Jean, Essay on Human Love (Rockcliff Publishing Co., 1951). p. 62.
14 Truffaut, François, The Wild Child, trans. Linda Lewin (New York: Washington Square Press, 1973), p. 12.
15 Allen, Don, François Truffaut (New York: The Viking Press, 1974); p. 56.
16 Truffaut, François, The Adventure of Antoine Doinel, trans. Helen G. Scott (New York: Simon and Schuster, 1971), p. 177.
17 Ibid., pp. 198–199.
18 Monaco, James, The New Wave (New York: Oxford University Press, 1976), pp. 43–44.
19 Crisp, C. G., François Truffaut (New York: Praeger, 1972), p. 118).
20 Truffaut, François, Jules and Jim (New York: Simon and Schuster. 1968), p. 19.
21 Ibid., p. 36.
22 Monaco, op. cit., p. 50.
23 Truffaut, François, Jules and Jim, p. 65.
24 Ibid., p. 59.
25 Crisp, op. cit., p. 63.

26 Allen, Don, op. cit., p. 154.
27 de Rougemont, Denis, Love Declared, p. 76.
28 Truffaut, François, The Story of Adele H. (New York: Grove Press.)
29 Ibid., p. 152.
30 A new film has been shown in France entitled L'Homme Qui Aimait Les Femmes, 1977.
31 Westerback, Collin, 'Fearful Symmetries', Commonweal, 27 February, 1976. p. 143.
32 Truffaut, François, Small Change (New York: Grove Press, 1976), p. 138.
33 Ibid., p. 157.
34 Ibid., p. 178.
35 Ibid., p. 187.
36 Truffaut, François, Adele H., p. 9.

IRA GROSS, Ph.D.

MENTAL HEALTH IN BOYS AND GIRLS: AWARENESS OF ATTITUDES FOR POSITIVE SEX ROLES

SUMMARY. The mental health of boys and girls can be improved through encouraging their awareness of socializing influences on their acquisition of sex roles. A complementary understanding needs to be developed in socializing agents as well. Psychologists and other social scientists have not facilitated this process — because of their own failure to address issues which underly both theory and practice. The reasons for this failure are considered and suggestions are presented for parents, educators, and social scientists to involve themselves meaningfully in the process of developing attitudes for positive sex roles.

IDEOLOGICAL BIAS IN THEORIES OF CHILD PSYCHOLOGY

It is not an indulgence to proceed with the task of promoting mental health by suggesting that social scientists need to heal themselves by increasing their awareness of the ideological biases in their theorizing about child psychology. The Year of the Child served to underscore the need for social scientists to be aware that theories about children are cultural inventions (Kessen, 1979). In the particular instance of role differentiated behavior it should be evident that social scientists have avoided confronting the influences which derive from politicization of theoretical constructs (Ingelby, 1974). This attitude has been managed by extirpating ideology from the main body of child psychology and concentrating it in topics on socialization (Harre, 1974). Sex role theory, as a specific instance of ideologizing, incorporates those prejudices in views which reflect 'appropriate' roles for each sex. Considered from this perspective the extant major theories ignore the ubiquitous influences that shape and define sex roles from the very earliest interactions between children and agents of socialization (Sears, Maccoby, and Levin, 1957).

The effects of ideologizing of sex roles on mental health may not be direct but they are insidiously pervasive. Such effects run counter-to several central values held by today's youth. Among these values are a striving for individuality and its expression through actualization of talents and interests. In order to realize these values young people must transcend many of the stereotyped expectations of society. Usually there is a price extracted for such transgression and it is often paid in the coin of distorted self-worth which is reinforced by the negative perceptions of such expressions by parents and other social agents. Thus, fulfillment of unique abilities and development of identity are encumbered by the proscriptions and imperatives of society.

If we are to promote mental health in our young people we must make conscious those aspects of ideology which circumscribe the freedom of choice and undermine the motivation to be interested in or strive for goals which may conflict with stereotypic expectations.

I. Gross, J. Downing, and A. d'Heurle (eds.), Sex Role Attitudes and Cultural Change, 197–200.
Copyright © 1982 by D. Reidel Publishing Company.

STUDENT PROGRAMS FOR AWARENESS AND SELF-DIRECTION

Of particular relevance for promoting healthy attitudes toward sex roles is the need to facilitate boys and girls self-direction. Such facilitation can come from two fundamental agents for socialization, parents and educators. Parents and educators can improve their contribution to this process by developing an organized program for addressing sex role attitudes. Basically, such a program has three principal components.

1. *Informational*: providing accurate information about the formation of attitudes about sex roles.

2. *Dialogue*: entering into a dialogue concerning the formation of attitudes and encouraging thereby exploration without imposition of preconceived notions.

3. *Policies and practices*: setting into practice policies which derive from the dialogue.

The initiation of this program presupposes corollary programs for parents and professionals. In order to undertake a program of change participants must be encouraged to question traditional stereotypes in sex roles and be willing to guide themselves toward a transformation of their attitudes. As a specific program of change in sex role attitudes the following general ideas should be addressed by parents and educators in the order presented.

PARENT AND EDUCATOR PROGRAMS FOR CHANGES IN SEX ROLE ATTITUDES

1. *Communicating and transmitting attitudes*: parents and educators need to be assisted toward a recognition of the reasons for considering changes in their means of communicating and transmitting attitudes which differentially encourage sex role behavior.

2. *Access to Information*: parents and educators need to have access to relevant information concerning sex role behavior. They need to know how such behavior develops and how as agents of socialization they can positively encourage the acquisition of healthy attitudes.

3. *Dialogue*: parents and educators need to develop the atmosphere and means for a dialogue with boys and girls regarding differences and similarities in sex role behavior.

Attitudes of Professionals

Professionals in mental health can contribute meaningfully in the aforementioned efforts if they, in turn, desist from the expositon of theories and practices retrogressive to the process. Ultimately parents and educators will look to theory in child psychology for encouragement and direction in their programs and practices. Should such theory be wanting in its contribution then very little change can be anticipated in attitude and in behavior. Therefore social scientists need to concern themselves with the sources of bias in theories about sex role and its development.

Issues Which Need to be Addressed

1. *Sex roles and biologizing*: there is sufficient evidence in human development to question the notion that sex roles embody biological universals. The trend of biologizing sex roles in the absence of empirical evidence (Lloyd, 1976) needs to be corrected by focussing on culture specific influences and their effects on attitudes and behavior.

2. *Forces which influence sex role expectations*: sex roles are products of the orientation of a society and as such are subject to the vagaries of change attendant upon historical, social, and economic needs. The effects of these influences need to be clarified with respect to culture specific sex role expectations.

3. *Similarities between the sexes*: much of the research on human sex roles has focused on the contrasts between behavior. What is clearly missing is an appropriate emphasis on understanding the similarities of psychological behavior between the sexes rather than just differences. Ultimately this can lead to complementarity through better relationships between the sexes.

CONCLUSIONS

The evidence and effects of sex role stereotyping have been amply documented with respect to both psychological theory and social practice (Maccoby and Jacklin, 1974). The need to redress the imbalances in interest and bias is self-evident. Parents, educators, and social scientists need to address the negative influences asserted by prevailing stereotypes. Professionals whose theories are merely descriptions of the status quo rather than explorations of possibilities for fulfillment simply endorse traditional shibboleths. Such descriptions need to be replaced by empirical studies documenting the salutary effects of self-actualization. It is suggested that one way to approach the need for change is to enter into a dialogue with youth which encourages exploration of issues and supports attempts at fulfillment which may be at odds with prevailing expectations. In addition social scientists need to concern themselves with the similarities between the sexes in order to facilitate the process of transcending traditional schisms and misunderstandings.

University of Rhode Island

REFERENCES

Clausen, J.
  1968 A historical and comparative view of socialization theory and research. In Clausen,
        J. (ed.)
Harre, R.
  1974 The conditions for a social psychology of childhood. In Richards, M. P. M. (eds.),
        The Integration of a Child into a Social World. London: Cambridge University
        Press.
Ingleby, D.
  1974 The psychology of child psychology. In Richards, M. P. M. (ed.), The Integration
        of a Child into a Social World. London: Cambridge University Press.
Kessen, W.
  1979 The American Child and Other Cultural Inventions. American Psychologist 34:
        815–820.
Lloyd, B.
  1976 Social responsibility and research on sex differences. In Lloyd, B. and Archer, J.
        (eds.), Exploring Sex Differences. London: Academic Press.
Maccobby, E. E. and Jacklin, C. N.
  1974 The Psychology of Sex Differences. Stanford: Stanford University Press.
Sears, R. R., E. E. Maccobby, and H. Levin
  1957 Patterns of Child Rearing. New York: Harper & Row.

IRA GROSS, Ph.D. and ADMA D'HEURLE, Ph.D.

DISCUSSION

The underlying concern expressed by participants in the two workshops spanning the World Congresses of 1977 and 1979 was for translating research on sex
roles into viable action for improving the development of mentally healthy males
and females. Among the more obvious reasons that such applications have not
been widely attempted are the cultural differences which affect action programs.
Such diversity, apparent in the presentations at these workshops, often impeded
general agreement as to significant issues, concepts and the emphasis required
for applications in different parts of the world. The single topic which did elicit
general agreement was the idea that prevailing biases constrained the development of healthy and creative persons. The nub of disagreement revolved around
the very means to encourage greater freedom for actualizing full individual
potential. The participants acknowledged the cultural differences and moved
toward agreement with respect to a stated position regarding the major goals
to be addressed in any effort at change while leaving open the means to achieve
these goals.

Among the topics discussed was the differential treatment accorded the
sexes in early childhood and throughout the school years. The school itself as
a powerful socializing agent came under close scrutiny. Among the different
aspects of school influence was the emphasis placed on the often opposing
roles of education as a conservative transmitter of values and tradition balanced
against the school's concern for innovation and change. Among the suggestions
made and reviewed, of recent attempts at change, were the development of
specific curricular materials and methods of instruction directed to encouraging a nonsexist understanding of life. One concern expressed was for the
insidious 'hidden curriculum' which promotes artificial barriers by segregating
the sexes.

The school's potential for correcting biases and the specific methods for
accomplishing this was discussed. Particular attention was given to the curriculum
itself and materials used in nonsexist approaches were presented. The value of
such materials was placed within the context of a fundamentally sound general
curriculum without which the goals of nonsexist education may be largely
irrelevant.

In addition to formal curricular materials the atmosphere of the schools was
identified as a crucial element for encouraging changes. Among the features of
school atmosphere was a willingness by educators to encourage dialogue in
several ways. The schools themselves must be prepared to facilitate discussion
with and among boys and girls, they must also be willing to include parents in
such discussions if any effective change can be expected to take place. Several

201

I. Gross, J. Downing, and A. d'Heurle (eds.), Sex Role Attitudes and Cultural Change, 201–203.
Copyright © 1982 by D. Reidel Publishing Company.

participants expressed such concerns in their respective presentations and in the ensuing discussions resulting from their comments.

Among other topics presented were the role perceptions of adult men and women and some changes in practices for family, marriage and occupational activity. Particular emphasis was given to the role of language and to the exclusionary terminology which prevails through the usage of masculine oriented gender generic language. By removing such traditional features of communication a healthier perception of role contribution is facilitated. Thus, selecting out terms such as 'fireman' and replacing it with 'fire-fighter' may seem a small – but recognizable incremental change in attitude which does not inadvertently place one gender at a disadvantage.

The effects of adult role perceptions on reproduction and family patterns were also discussed at some length. Some apprehension was expressed about the acceptance of nontraditional ways of defining the place of reproduction and of parenting in human experience. In part this disagreement was resolved by accepting a position which recognizes and promotes alternative attitudes and practices to the extent that they recognize the value of the individual and provide a greater margin for individual choice.

Considerable time was devoted to discussing the place of the scientific study of sex differences and here opinions diverged sharply. Some workshop members expressed the view that scientific evidence about sex differences is the only valid basis for discussing potential changes in policies and programs. Others believed that to date scientific studies have placed inordinate weight on the differences between the sexes and have not balanced this with due consideration of the congruences and similarities between the sexes. It was strongly urged that the topics of child care methods, educational programs and relations between the sexes must proceed from existing scientific knowledge about socialization while also showing regard for the cultural context of which they are part. Here as in other topics discussed the role of scientific knowledge in promoting healthy attitudes proved to be inconclusive.

As a group the members of the workshop became convinced of the value of continuing their efforts through future World Congresses. The goals they hoped to achieve through such efforts were: to deepen the participants understanding of sex role and culture; to communicate the insights and understanding gained from this experience to a wider audience; and as professionals to work actively towards the goal of equality between the sexes. Disagreements notwithstanding the participants did recognize that mental health could be promoted through existing knowledge and evidence in specific ways. Among the ways to encourage positive mental health and the development of such attitudes at all ages the following set of guidelines are seen as facilitative: setting standards for appropriate attitudes and behavior in diverse contexts, such as the school, occupations, and interpersonal relations; providing appropriate role models and as professionals demonstrating such modeling through their own behavior; enhancing equal opportunities for both sexes; changing and shaping attitudes and practices; and finally by promoting a humanistic dialogue regarding sex roles.

It is abundantly clear that the World Congress has served an important role in providing the platform for exchange of professional ideas, research and attitudes about mental health and sex roles. Rather than detracting from the value of the topic, the diversity of opinions and positions attests to the viability of the theme and the uncertain state of current knowledge. It is no small wonder that agreements may be too few when one considers the intransigence of attitudes and practices surrounding this topic. Discussion and research will continue to evolve and sharp debate should help to overcome conceptual shortcomings. It was generally agreed that as more empirical data accrues this will also serve to clarify issues and direct efforts with greater certainty toward goals of improved mental health and promote greater understanding of the means for changing sex role attitudes. As yet we are still at the cross roads and with incomplete maps to guide us we steer a course through uncharted waters. All of the participants agreed that the voyage was worth understanding even if the destination seemed distant and elusive.

University of Rhode Island (I. G.)
Mercy College, Dobbs Ferry, New York (A. d'H.)

INDEX OF NAMES

INDEX OF SUBJECTS